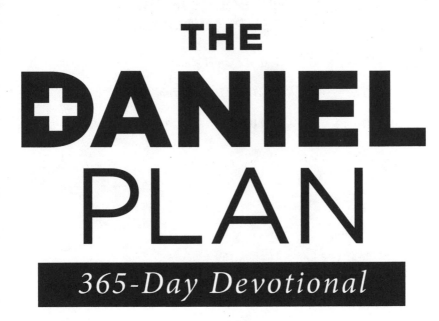

THE
✝DANIEL
PLAN

365-Day Devotional

OTHER BOOKS IN THE DANIEL PLAN SERIES:

The Daniel Plan

The Daniel Plan Journal

The Daniel Plan Cookbook

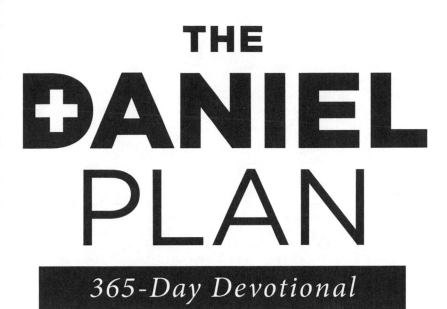

THE
ÐANIEL
PLAN

365-Day Devotional

DAILY ENCOURAGEMENT
for a HEALTHIER LIFE

A COMPANION TO THE #1 NEW YORK TIMES BESTSELLER,
THE DANIEL PLAN: 40 DAYS TO A HEALTHIER LIFE

THE DANIEL PLAN TEAM

With DEE EASTMAN
& KAREN LEE-THORP

INTRODUCTION BY RICK WARREN

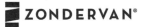
ZONDERVAN®

ZONDERVAN

The Daniel Plan 365-Day Devotional
Copyright © 2015 by The Daniel Plan

This title is also available as a Zondervan ebook.
Visit www.zondervan.com/ebooks.

Requests for information should be addressed to:
Zondervan, 3900 *Sparks Dr. SE, Grand Rapids, Michigan 49546*

Library of Congress Cataloging-in-Publication Data

ISBN 978-0-310-34563-3

Published in association with Josh Warren, RKW Legacy Partners, 29881 Santa Margarita Parkway, Rancho Santa Margarita, CA 92688

Art direction: Curt Diepenhorst
Interior design: Kait Lamphere

First printing August 2015 / Printed in the United States of America

INTRODUCTION

I'm so thankful for your continued commitment to The Daniel Plan. It's hard work to get healthy, but it's worth it because the benefits aren't just physical; they're also eternal! When you're physically healthy, you have more energy and strength to do what God wants you to do with your life.

The Daniel Plan isn't about counting calories. It's about achieving health in every area of your life. That's why I want to make sure you're focusing on all five Essentials of the Daniel Plan food and fitness, but also faith, focus, and friends.

You've probably already realized in your journey to get healthy that if you want to make lasting changes in your life, you need the right support. That's why I asked Dee Eastman and Karen Lee-Thorp to write devotionals that will encourage you every day.

These devotionals will equip you to face the ups and downs that come with living a healthy lifestyle, and they will help you draw deeply from a daily quiet time with God. Each day you'll find a key verse from God's Word, inspiration that builds on the theme of the day, application to your own life, and some "Food for Thought" to nourish you.

My prayer for you is "that you may enjoy good health and that all may go well with you, even as your soul is getting along well" (3 John 1:2). I believe that God will bless you spiritually and physically through these devotionals and that one year from today, you will be healthier and you will have accomplished your Daniel Plan goals with this daily encouragement.

You're on the right track to the abundant life full of energy and purpose God intended for you.

Keep going!

Rick Warren

NEW YEAR, NEW YOU

See, I am doing a new thing! Now it springs up; do you not perceive it? I am making a way in the wilderness and streams in the wasteland.

—Isaiah 43:19

A new year is a time to start fresh. No matter what your history is with faith, food, fitness, focus, or friends, this is a great day to turn a new page. If you've had areas of wasteland in your life, God wants to pour streams into that desert and make it bloom. Nothing is impossible for him. He says, "I am the LORD, the God of all mankind. Is anything too hard for me?" (Jeremiah 32:27). The answer is no.

With this new year, set some goals for yourself. Goals are the steps we take each day, week, and month to get from where we are today to the future we dream of having. A goal is a dream with a deadline. If you knew you couldn't fail, what would you like to do with your life this year? What is one goal you'd like to start with, knowing that it's up to God to make it possible?

FOOD FOR THOUGHT

God is doing a new thing in you. He's making a way for you to walk toward the life he has in store for you.

SAY NO TO SAY YES

The king assigned them a daily amount of food and wine from the king's table.... But Daniel resolved not to defile himself with the royal food and wine, and he asked the chief official for permission not to defile himself this way.
—Daniel 1:5, 8

D aniel was a captive in a pagan country, a young man forced to serve another country's government. He obediently went into their training program but insisted on eating only food that was kosher under Jewish law. This was an essential part of his Jewish faith—and essential to operate at his best. He had the courage to stand up to his captors, even though they didn't understand his commitment, and to seek an arrangement that would satisfy them without defiling himself.

When we commit ourselves to The Daniel Plan lifestyle, we will sometimes have to say no to an old way of living in order to say yes to caring for the body and soul God has given us. We're saying yes to abundance, yes to health, and yes to having the energy to serve him. What will you say yes to today?

FOOD FOR THOUGHT

Sometimes we need to say no to something in order to say yes to God.

GOD'S MASTERPIECE

For we are God's handiwork, created in Christ Jesus to do good works,
which God prepared in advance for us to do.   —*Ephesians 2:10*

Imagine being God's masterpiece, his priceless work of art, unlike any other. That's your value: priceless. Your value doesn't come from the clothes you wear, a number on a scale, your career, or your success with a health plan on any given day. You are of immense value because God made you. If that's not enough, Jesus died for you and the Holy Spirit lives in you. As unbelievable as it sounds, doubting your value is actually unbelief in his Word. What would you do differently if you were sure you were of immense value?

Doing good deeds and making good choices doesn't make you more valuable to God. Instead, doing good things flows out of the value you already have. God made you to do things that only you could do. If you don't know what those good things are, start with what you know. Offer to do something at your church or in your community. Reach out to a friend. Ask God to show you the good things you were made to do.

FOOD FOR THOUGHT

Only you can make the contribution to this world for which God has uniquely and wonderfully made you.

LET THE SPIRIT RENEW YOU

Be made new in the attitude of your minds.

—*Ephesians 4:23*

Thoughts and attitudes are important because they determine what you feel. Thoughts, attitudes, and feelings then determine what you do. Some of your thoughts are on the surface of your mind, and you're aware of them. But some of your thoughts and attitudes are rooted deep down in your heart, and you're seldom consciously aware of them.

I'll never change.

I've been like this my whole life.

I can't do it.

I'm too busy.

When thoughts like these well up from deep inside us, they block us from doing the things God wants us to do.

What can we do about these thoughts that have been rooted inside us for years? We must invite the Holy Spirit to expose them so that we're consciously aware of them. Then we can ask, "Is it true?" That's a crucial question about any thought that is an obstacle to change. Then the Holy Spirit will help us uproot thoughts that aren't true. He is eager to help. Ask him.

FOOD FOR THOUGHT

Ask the Holy Spirit to reveal the deep-rooted negative thoughts that stand in the way of your transformation.

PURE DELIGHT

They delight in the law of the Lord, meditating on it day and night.
—Psalm 1:2 NLT

The psalmist speaks of the person who is blessed, fortunate, and happy. He meditates on God's Word day and night. To meditate is to think deeply about something, to go over and over it so that it sinks into the heart and influences the way we think, feel, and act.

Repetition helps us create habits and can transform us. Just as repeatedly eating the right foods or consistently exercising changes our bodies over time, so repeating a passage of Scripture and consistently thinking about it will gradually change the way we think. And changing the way we think will change the way we live.

Choose a verse that ministers to your soul, perhaps a promise you want to trust in. Turn it over and over in your mind. What are the implications of it? Let it sink into your heart.

FOOD FOR THOUGHT

If you can make space to meditate daily on a short portion of God's Word, you will change your mind-set and your heart over time.

A GOD-FASHIONED LIFE

*Whatever is true, whatever is noble, whatever is right, whatever is pure,
whatever is lovely, whatever is admirable—if anything is excellent or
praiseworthy—think about such things.* —Philippians 4:8

Pastor Rick Warren says, "The way you think determines the way you feel, and the way you feel determines the way you act." If we want to change any behavior, we must start by challenging unhealthy perspectives. The Daniel Plan requires a new attitude. Being made new like this begins when we challenge our distorted ways of thinking. We ask, "Is that right? Does that fit with God's Word and God's wisdom? Or did somebody somewhere tell me that, but it simply isn't true?"

Pastor Warren also says, "We must make healthy choices to use the resources God has given us, and the first healthy choice is to be careful about what we think." So what are you thinking about today?

Think about what is true—what is true about God, what is true about your identity in Christ, and about the promises of God.

FOOD FOR THOUGHT

How powerful it can be when we challenge our unhealthy perspectives and replace them with God's truth.

DETOX

Let us purify ourselves from everything that contaminates body and spirit,
perfecting holiness out of reverence for God.   —2 Corinthians 7:1

What contaminates the spirit? Anything that takes our eyes off Christ. When Paul spoke of these things, he probably was referring to sexual sin, but certainly our bodies need to be purified from things we eat or drink that aren't good for us, too. We need to detox from all of it.

To "detox" means to rid ourselves of toxic substances. We detox from artificial, manmade foods out of reverence for God—out of the knowledge that God made our bodies and wants us to care for them. We detox so that we can enjoy the abundance of foods God created to nourish us. Detoxing is about abundance, not deprivation, because the foods we are saying no to aren't really foods at all.

As Dr. Mark Hyman says, "The best thing you can do for your health is to avoid factory-made science projects that haven't been made by God in nature." Emphasize bringing in the array of delicious, replenishing foods that God made for your pleasure and well-being.

FOOD FOR THOUGHT

God has made an abundance of good and flavor-rich foods for our enjoyment, so purifying our bodies can actually be fulfilling and satisfying.

ULTIMATELY SAFE

*My God sent his angel, and he shut the mouths of the lions. They have not
hurt me, because I was found innocent in his sight.* —Daniel 6:22

Daniel continued his habit of prayer to God even when prayer was
outlawed, so the king of Persia had him thrown into a den of
lions. God prevented the lions from killing Daniel in order to show
the king that God really was God and Daniel was his innocent servant.

God doesn't always shut the mouths of the lions. Sometimes bad
situations happen to his loyal servants. But nothing can *ultimately*
harm those who are faithful to him. We are safe from all enemies and
even from death because God will raise us from the dead. Knowing
this, we can face the lions with the same courage as Daniel.

The psalmist says, "My heart is glad and my tongue rejoices; my
body also will rest secure" (Psalm 16:9). How bold and confident will
you be about your faith, knowing you are safe in his loving arms?

FOOD FOR THOUGHT

Don't let fear get in the way; God always goes
before you.

IDENTIFYING PASSION

The Holy Spirit is given to each of us in a special way. That is for the good of all.
— *1 Corinthians 12:7 NIrV*

God has given us the Holy Spirit so we can make unique contributions to the world. You may not have one mission for your whole life, and you don't need to know what God plans for you to do twenty years from now. What you need to know is what God wants of you in this season. How has God shaped you to contribute to his world here and now?

God designed us to have passion. We are supposed to feel things. Passion helps us move ahead, have energy, and persevere through conflicts. We know we have passion when we lose track of time while doing something. What are those things that you enjoy so much that you forget the time?

If you don't know what you're passionate about, experiment with different activities until you find one that lights you up. Frederick Buechner said, "The place God calls you to is the place where your deep gladness and the world's deep hunger meet."[1]

FOOD FOR THOUGHT

When the Holy Spirit and your passion come together, you have a powerful opportunity to make a difference in the world.

FOCUS ON GOD'S PRIORITIES

You make known to me the path of life; you will fill me with joy in your presence, with eternal pleasures at your right hand. —Psalm 16:11

So many distractions compete for our attention. We need to focus on God's plans and priorities for our lives. Some of those priorities are the same for every person: seeking God's kingdom, loving our neighbors. Some priorities are unique to the stage of life we are in. Consider taking some time to think through the top priorities in your life. What does God want you to be devoted to at this point?

Does taking care of your spiritual, emotional, and physical health make it onto your list? If you give careful attention to those, you'll have the energy to fulfill everything else God has called you to do.

God wants you to experience the fullness of joy. You can do that by drawing near to him and letting him show you the path of your life. Try not to let distractions pull you away from that path; it's the one that leads to eternal joy.

FOOD FOR THOUGHT

Choosing God's path for you will lead you to fullness of joy.

MOVEMENT THAT FEELS LIKE PLAY

Let them praise his name with dancing and make music to him with timbrel and harp. —*Psalm 149:3*

How are you doing at discovering movement you enjoy, movement that feels like play to you? There's a saying that goes, "We do not quit playing because we grow old; we grow old because we quit playing." We are designed to take joy in our bodies' ability to move in so many different ways. The ancient Israelites even praised God with dancing.

If you've been doing the same kind of movement for some time, perhaps it's time to bring some variety to your workouts. Fitness expert Sean Foy says, "Changing your scenery, meeting new people, and trying something different can be just what you need to keep your fitness routine fresh."

You're not on this fitness journey alone. God is with you to keep you steady and on track. Consider thanking and praising him as you move your body. Ask him to help you discover movement you can feel passionate about.

FOOD FOR THOUGHT

God wants to help you get to a place where movement is playful and full of joy, celebrating him.

MORE SOLID THAN MOUNTAINS

Even if the mountains walk away and the hills fall to pieces, my love won't walk away from you. —*Isaiah 54:10 MSG*

Do you find it hard to believe the depth of God's love? If it's hard for you to reach out in love to other people, it may be that you are not secure in knowing that you are unconditionally loved. If you are secure in God's love for you, his acceptance can help you handle the imperfect ways of other people. You can concentrate on loving them and not worry too much if they don't make you feel deeply loved in return.

Meditate on this truth: God's love for you is more solid than a mountain. Mountains are slowly worn down by rain, wind, sun, and snow, but nothing wears down God's love. No earthquake will shake his love. Nothing bad you've done, no personality quirk or limitation of yours can undermine his absolute delight in you just the way you are. Let his love enrich your life and the lives of those around you.

FOOD FOR THOUGHT

Picture a mountain. God's love for you is much taller and wider, and he promises that his love will never fail.

EYES ON JESUS

Let us keep looking to Jesus. He is the one who started this journey of faith.
And he is the one who completes the journey of faith.

—*Hebrews 12:2 NIrV*

If you want your mind to be healthy, focus your thoughts on what is true and good. Nothing is truer or better than Jesus. Study how he lived, because his life is the one to imitate. Read the Gospels, which tell the story of his life. Ask yourself, what did Jesus do that I could learn from? Picture him running the race just ahead of you, showing you how it's done.

During his earthly life, Jesus focused his thoughts beyond the cross to the joy waiting for him in the Father's presence. Focusing on that joy at the finish line enabled him to put up with anything during the race—even when people didn't respond to him with faith and love. He spent plenty of time alone with his Father, so people didn't keep him down. When the road seems difficult, ask him to guide and strengthen you.

FOOD FOR THOUGHT

Keep your eyes on Jesus, and you'll find you are able to overcome anything that stands in your way.

GUARD YOUR HEART

Above all else, guard your heart, for everything you do flows from it.

—*Proverbs 4:23*

When the proverb says, "Guard your heart," it means "Guard the part of you where your deepest, most fundamental thoughts and beliefs are stored." That's what the heart signified in ancient Hebrew culture. The reason for guarding these deepest thoughts is because they determine how you feel, what you do, and therefore, how your life goes. If your deepest attitudes are distorted, your life will reflect that. But if the deep beliefs that motivate you are true and good, your life will flourish.

We are usually most interested in God changing our circumstances, taking away our suffering. But God is most interested in changing our hearts and actions. That's because who you are and will be for all eternity is shaped primarily not by what happens to you, but by how you respond to what happens to you. And how you respond is shaped by what you think deep down in your heart. So feed your heart plenty of true, good, and lovely things (Philippians 4:8), and guard what goes on in it.

FOOD FOR THOUGHT

Your heart is the wellspring from which your life flows. Guard it well.

THE GIFT OF SLEEP

I lie down and sleep; I wake again, because the Lord sustains me.

—*Psalm 3:5*

Sleep is the ultimate form of trusting God. Going to sleep means letting go of control over the world, trusting God to take care of things while we're unconscious. We trust God to sustain us while we sleep.

We need sleep to be effective so we can be focused when we're awake. People who get less than six or seven hours of sleep at night have lower blood flow to the brain, which leads to poorer decision-making ability. Dr. Daniel Amen says getting inadequate sleep turns off 700 health-promoting genes. Therefore, sometimes the healthiest and most spiritual thing you can do is to go to bed.

Sleep is God's gift to us. The Bible says, *"God gives rest to his loved ones"* (Psalm 127:2 NLT). If you're not getting enough sleep, look closely at your schedule and ask God what activities or worries you need to re-evaluate or let go.

FOOD FOR THOUGHT

Sleep is a blessing God gives to refresh and replenish us. Have you accepted this gift?

RECOVERING YOUR JOY

Restore to me the joy of your salvation.

—*Psalm 51:12*

Think of a time in your life when you had joy, the kind that comes from knowing the Father loves you, Jesus died for you, and the Holy Spirit lives inside you. Where is that joy today? Has it been stolen by daily hassles or a loss? If so, God wants to restore your joy. It may not happen at the snap of a finger, but you can discover joy in God even when life is far from perfect.

The first step in recovering joy is believing that God wants you to have it. The next step is asking for it. Why not make that prayer the desire of your heart, something you take to God regularly?

The third step is to draw near to him. There is so much joy in sitting before him, letting him love you in spite of circumstances, experiencing anew the gift of his presence in your life.

The fourth step is to choose to set your mind on things that foster joy. What people, activities, websites, books, and entertainment foster joy in you, and which ones deplete your joy? Take your pick.

FOOD FOR THOUGHT

God is eager to give you joy as you bask in his presence.

CHANGING YOUR MIND

"Repent, for the kingdom of heaven has come near."

—Matthew 4:17

The Greek word for repentance, *metanoia*, means changing one's mind. It's not just the shifting of an opinion or action, but a deep change in thoughts and attitudes that leads to total reorientation. Our orientation toward sin changes to an orientation toward God, from our way to God's way. This can start with a one-time decision, but it plays out every day.

Daily time in God's Word is essential to this ongoing process. For example, we might sit down to read with no notion that we even need to change something. Then the Word challenges us with a new idea. Now we are thinking about the possibility of change. We may or may not be different overnight, but the Word lifts us out of denial and out of rationalizing our actions into questioning them and entertaining a new way of thinking. Now it will take courage to put that new thinking into action. Thankfully, that's the Holy Spirit's job.

Repent today, and dive into God's Word.

FOOD FOR THOUGHT

God will reorient our lives as we expose our minds to the truths of Scripture.

THE GOD WHO SEES YOU

*She gave this name to the L*ORD *who spoke to her: "You are the God who sees me."*
—Genesis 16:13

Hagar was a slave woman who belonged to Abraham and Sarah, a childless couple who wanted a son. According to the laws of the day, if Abraham had a child with Hagar, it would be legally Abraham and Sarah's child. Sarah talked Abraham into taking that route. But when Hagar got pregnant, she sneered at Sarah, and Sarah drove Hagar to run away. After being used and abused, Hagar was resting beside a spring in the desert when the Lord reassured her that he was looking out for her and her unborn son. Astonished, she called him "the God who sees me."

No matter what your circumstances are, the Lord sees you. He sees everything that happens to you, and he cares. He is looking out for you the way he looked out for Hagar.

FOOD FOR THOUGHT

God sees you as you are, everything about you and everything that happens to you. He is right by your side.

THE LORD'S BATTLE

*"It is not by sword or spear that the Lord saves; for the battle is the Lord's,
and he will give all of you into our hands."*   —1 Samuel 17:47

Teenage David defeated gigantic Goliath with a slingshot and a few stones. But before he overcame Goliath, he overcame an even bigger enemy: discouragement. First from his older brother, then from King Saul, and finally from Goliath himself. All of them said David couldn't do it.

David persevered not because he believed in himself but because he believed in God. Your goals for getting healthy do not depend solely on you. Turn them over to God, and let him wage the battle for you.

If you are ever feeling discouraged, think of what David was able to do with his slingshot. Picture him standing up to the people who said it couldn't be done. Pray for courage like David's. God will empower you as you trust in him. You will be able to say, like David, "This is the Lord's battle."

FOOD FOR THOUGHT

If you have been visited by discouragement, don't let it stand in your way. God is ready to accompany you into battle.

A NEW WAY TO THINK

*Be merciful to me, Lord, for I am in distress.... I am forgotten as though
I were dead; I have become like broken pottery.*   —Psalm 31:9, 12

Ever feel like everything is against you? Or like you are stuck in negative thought patterns? One pattern to watch out for is overgeneralization. This usually involves words like *always, never, every time,* or *everyone.* These thoughts make a situation out to be worse than it really is.

For instance, "I have always struggled with health issues; it will never change" or "Every time I get stressed, I fall into bad patterns." Are these thoughts accurate? Do you know it will *never* change? Do you *have to* fall into bad patterns every time, without exception? Of course not. Overgeneralizations make you believe you have no control over your actions and that you are incapable of changing them.

If you tend to think in overgeneralizations, write them down and challenge them. Then turn your heart to what you know is true: the power of the Holy Spirit is within you.

FOOD FOR THOUGHT

God is merciful; he will free you from those old thought patterns.

EVEN IF HE DOES NOT

"If we are thrown into the blazing furnace, the God we serve is able to deliver us from it . . . But even if he does not . . . we will not serve your gods or worship the image of gold you have set up." —Daniel 3:17–18

Three friends were under threat of death if they refused to worship an idol. They had faith that God was able to protect them from the death sentence, but *even if God didn't do what they wanted*, they were committed to him. They were committed because they were confident that he knew what was best in the big picture of his plan for the world. They counted their lives as worthy of sacrifice for God.

What do you long for God to do for you? He is able to do it. He is a good, loving, wise, and all-powerful God. He calls you to trust him. Can you honestly say, "I know God can come through for me on this, *and even if he doesn't*, I am wholly committed to him"? Depend on him; he will do what is best, and you are part of that plan.

FOOD FOR THOUGHT

No matter what life brings, we have a God who is worthy of our trust.

PREDICTING THE FUTURE

If you say, "The LORD is my refuge," and you make the Most High your dwelling, no harm will overtake you, no disaster will come near your tent.
—Psalm 91:9–10

One harmful form of negative thinking is predicting the worst in a situation. Predicting the worst immediately throws you into anxiety. Anxiety can lead you to turn to comfortable but unhealthy habits—you need to eat sugar or zone out in front of the TV just to calm your nerves. Plus, if you envision and expect the worst, your mind tends to make it happen.

For example, "Healthy food will be expensive, taste like cardboard, and won't fill me up." Are you sure of that? How do you know if you haven't even tried the meal plan? Or "I won't be able to finish this project on time." Are your expectations making failure more likely? Are they causing anxiety that slows down your thinking and progress?

Instead of predicting the worst, consider entrusting your fears to God and stepping out in faith. The worst that will happen is probably not as bad as the horrible future you've predicted.

FOOD FOR THOUGHT

Instead of predicting the worst, make the Lord your refuge. If you dwell in him, you can expect he will always be right by your side.

THE BLAME GAME

The man said, "The woman you put here with me—she gave me some
fruit from the tree, and I ate it." —Genesis 3:12

When Adam ate the forbidden fruit and the Lord questioned him about it, he immediately blamed Eve rather than taking responsibility for his actions. We do this too sometimes, blaming others for the problems in our lives.

"My unhealthy habits are my parents' fault; this is how they raised me."

"I'm overweight because of my genetics."

"The reason I'm stuck in this bad mood is because you keep picking at me."

Blaming will never get us anywhere. It makes us the victims of other people or circumstances, as though we can't do anything to change the situation. In reality, though, there is something we can do.

The first step out of the blame game is to question the blaming thought. Is this truly 100 percent the fault of the other person, my genetics, or my circumstances? How have I contributed to this situation? How would God enable me to do something differently? He is eager to empower us to break free from old patterns.

FOOD FOR THOUGHT

Stop blaming someone or something else for your problems. You have more power than you know.

JOY DESPITE SUFFERING

Though the fig tree does not bud and there are no grapes on the vines, though the olive crop fails and the fields produce no food, though there are no sheep in the pen and no cattle in the stalls, yet I will rejoice in the LORD, I will be joyful in God my Savior. —Habakkuk 3:17–18

Anybody can be joyful if circumstances are going well. The real test is whether we can be like Habakkuk, rejoicing that God is our Savior even when life is heartbreaking and God seems silent.

It's natural to pay more attention to a broken arm than to all the parts of our bodies that aren't broken. We're hardwired to do that. Unfortunately, this trait makes us prone to focus on whatever is going wrong in our lives rather than on the solid truths about God that haven't changed.

If you've been swamped by negative circumstances, take some time out and think about God being your Savior, healer, and redeemer. No matter what obstacles are in your path, he promises the gift of his presence and the comfort of his never-ending love.

FOOD FOR THOUGHT

Rejoice because God is your Savior and his mercies are new every morning.

THE SILVER LINING, NOT THE CLOUD

Now I take limitations in stride, and with good cheer, these limitations that cut me down to size—abuse, accidents, opposition, bad breaks. I just let Christ take over! And so the weaker I get, the stronger I become.
—2 Corinthians 12:10 MSG

Some of us are masterful at finding something negative to say about any situation. This negative thinking takes a positive experience and taints it. Every silver lining has a cloud.

For instance, "I wanted to get two hours more sleep a night, but I've only managed one hour. I'm a complete failure."

What? This thought turns what was a good start into a big fail. However, by reframing it with a truthful, positive spin, we can actually make our brains release positive neurotransmitters that will help us keep making healthy choices. For example, "I am already getting an additional hour of sleep and have changed my lifestyle, so I will continue making changes until I reach my goal of eight hours each night." Isn't that a better way to take limitations "with good cheer," as the apostle Paul says? With Christ's help, those limitations won't have the last word.

FOOD FOR THOUGHT

You will see even more healthy changes in your life if you learn to celebrate what is positive instead of focusing on the negative.

CULTIVATING STILLNESS

"Be still, and know that I am God; I will be exalted among the nations,
I will be exalted in the earth."   *—Psalm 46:10*

S tudies have shown that prayer improves attention and planning, reduces depression and anxiety, decreases sleepiness, and protects the brain from cognitive decline associated with normal aging.[2] Making requests of God is one important form of prayer—he says to keep on asking and you shall receive (Luke 11:9).

Another essential type of prayer is to quiet yourself and focus your thoughts on the greatness and power of God. He is God. He is all-powerful, all-wise, all-loving. He is here with you right now, waiting for you to become aware of his presence. He knows all your needs, and there's nothing you need more than him.

Be still and meditate on these truths about him. Let your body relax into that awareness. Rest in his presence. Slow down your breathing. Exalt him. He is God.

If you have trouble just sitting in his presence, try repeating a verse of Scripture in your mind. Start with Psalm 46:10.

FOOD FOR THOUGHT

In the stillness, you will find rest and God will rejuvenate your heart and soul.

GOD'S POWER, NOT WILLPOWER

I can do all this through him who gives me strength.

—*Philippians 4:13*

What positive changes in your life could happen if you relied on God's unlimited power instead of your limited willpower? That's what faith is: doing God's will by God's power instead of on your own. God will help you as you rely on him to give you the ability to change what he wants you to change.

God understands you better than you understand yourself. God knows what makes you tick—he knows what energizes you, what fatigues you, what makes you sick, what makes you operate at your best. Doesn't it make sense to trust him to help you?

Without God's power in your life, you are like a laptop that is unplugged; the battery will eventually drain and shut down the computer. Why live like that? God created you for so much more.

When you think about change, don't limit yourself to only the changes you know you can make on your own. Dream of what you can become when God empowers you.

FOOD FOR THOUGHT

God wants to bring about amazing changes in your life.

THE GIFT OF GRATITUDE

Rejoice always, pray continually, give thanks in all circumstances; for this is God's will for you in Christ Jesus. —*1 Thessalonians 5:16–18*

Is it truly possible to give thanks in all circumstances? Yes. There might be aspects of the circumstance that God doesn't want— troubles caused by sin or the brokenness of a fallen world. But there are bound to be elements of the circumstance you can be thankful for. Thank God that he is with you. Thank him for how he can form your heart as you persevere. Thank him for helping you respond with love, faith, and hope. Thank him for the other people who are standing with you. Thank him for what he might be doing in their lives that you aren't aware of.

Once you get started, you can probably think of many more reasons to thank him. Write down these things instead of just thinking of them. Writing your gratitude helps to solidify it in your mind so that it affects your mood and your choices. Even better: tell someone else you are grateful for him or her for something specific. Spread the gratitude around.

FOOD FOR THOUGHT

Giving thanks in all circumstances will transform the way you experience your life and see the goodness of God.

ENCOURAGE ONE ANOTHER

Encourage one another and build each other up.

—*1 Thessalonians 5:11*

D o you want a relationship to turn toward a more positive direction? Write down at least three things you are grateful for about the other person. Then put one of those things in a note or text, and send it to the person. Or say it face to face. The other person will likely respond with happy surprise to being thanked. Even if he or she doesn't, you've still done something good.

Afterward, watch for more things you are grateful for in that person. Instead of noticing the negative part of an interaction, draw your attention to the positive, and thank the person for it. You will feel better about yourself, bless the other person, and revolutionize the relationship.

Try the same thing in your small group, if you have one: send texts of thanks to group members. Be specific about what you appreciate. You don't have to be the group leader to become the official encourager. Think how uplifted people will be to have someone in their lives who says thank you.

FOOD FOR THOUGHT

Today, change your whole mind-set by giving the gift of thankfulness to those around you.

PERSISTENT PRAYER

When Daniel learned that the decree had been published... Three times a day he got down on his knees and prayed, giving thanks to his God, just as he had done before. —Daniel 6:10

D aniel was a government official in Persia when a law against prayer to God was passed. The law carried the death sentence, but Daniel continued to pray, thank, and praise God three times a day. What a wonderful model Daniel gives us for a heart wholly devoted to God!

Why not try out Daniel's rhythm of prayer? Check in with God first thing in the morning; ask him to guide you in doing his will. Check in again around noon to thank him for the first half of the day and evaluate how you're doing with following his guidance. Then thank and praise him at the end of the day. Even if you can't stick perfectly to this routine every day, commit to grow in your relationship with God, and schedule times to regularly pray and listen to him. Just a few minutes here and there during a busy day can make an enormous difference in your dedication to him.

FOOD FOR THOUGHT

Find a rhythm of prayer that works for you. God delights when we regularly meet him in prayer.

WHY WE DON'T GIVE UP

Therefore we do not lose heart. Though outwardly we are wasting away, yet inwardly we are being renewed day by day. For our light and momentary troubles are achieving for us an eternal glory that far outweighs them all. —2 Corinthians 4:16–17

The apostle Paul gave two reasons why he didn't give up. Even though he acknowledged the limitations of his body, that didn't make him quit. Why not?

First, no matter how our bodies feel, our spirits are being renewed every day if we are in contact with God. If your spirit isn't being renewed, you may not be taking full advantage of connecting with God through prayer. His arms are open wide as he waits to receive you.

Second, our present troubles are small and won't last long. Now, Paul had enemies who wanted to kill him. He traveled hundreds of miles on foot, over roads with thieves, terrible weather, and wild animals. Yet he said his troubles were small. Why? Because he compared them to the glory ahead that vastly outweighed his earthly hardships. In that light, could your troubles be called small too?

FOOD FOR THOUGHT

Keeping our eyes focused on God will shrink our problems down to size.

LAUGHTER IS GOOD MEDICINE

A cheerful disposition is good for your health; gloom and doom leave you bone-tired. —*Proverbs 17:22 MSG*

Laughter is good for you. It lowers the flow of dangerous stress hormones in your body, eases digestion, and soothes stomachaches, a common symptom of chronic stress. So if you are under stress, consider relaxing with a comedy instead of a drama. Even better, spend some time with friends who bring out the lighter side of life.

If laughter doesn't come easily to you, ask yourself why that is the case. One possibility is that you're holding on to your worries instead of entrusting them to God. "Cast all your anxiety on him because he cares for you" (1 Peter 5:7).

Another possibility is that you're grieving a loss. There's a time for grief, and it's healthy to grieve. Be sure you're in a process of working through your grief with the help of others, and giving yourself grace in the process. Friends and entertainment that give you a break from sorrow might even be helpful as you move through grief.

Otherwise, find out what pokes your funny bone, and let it ease your stress.

FOOD FOR THOUGHT

Laughter truly is good medicine for the body and the soul.

BEATING BURNOUT

"I have had enough, LORD," [Elijah] said. "Take my life; I am no better than my ancestors."
                                                    —*1 Kings 19:4*

The prophet Elijah was one of the greatest prophets of all time. But at one point in his long labor of resisting Israel's evil queen, he got burned out. He told the Lord, "I quit."

The Lord knew what he needed. First, Elijah needed rest. The Lord gave him time to sleep, and then an angel woke him to offer some food he needed to eat and water he needed to drink. Often the solution to burnout is as simple as that: rest, nourishment, and hydration.

Elijah needed more. He needed some alone time with God. He traveled forty days and nights to get there. He had to get far away from the place where he labored to a place where he could be still and at peace. And God met him there, in that alone place. They had a bluntly honest talk. God renewed Elijah's soul. Then he honored God and went back to work filled up.

What do you need? Rest? Food? Water? Time with God?

FOOD FOR THOUGHT

Sometimes it's as simple as pouring yourself a cup of water and letting God quench your thirst.

TELLING THE TRUTH

Let us tell our neighbors the truth, for we are all parts of the same body.
—*Ephesians 4:25 NLT*

In order to change and get healthy, we all need at least one friend to whom we can tell the truth. A small group of friends is even better. These are the people with whom we go beyond, "I'm fine" and "Life's great." They are the ones we can trust to hear our struggles. These are the ones the proverb speaks of: "A friend loves at all times, and a brother is born for a time of adversity" (Proverbs 17:17).

We all struggle. God wants to meet you in the struggle. One of the ways he will do that is through a few trusted people who have demonstrated that they can handle the truth about you. Your areas of difficulty, the things you most want to hide from everyone else, are exactly what you most need to talk about with a trusted friend. Who is one person you can tell the truth to? What is the truth you need to tell?

FOOD FOR THOUGHT

Life really is better together—for a cord of three strands (you, a close friend, and God) is not easily broken.

THE GOODNESS OF REPENTANCE

*"The time has come," [Jesus] said. "The kingdom of God has come near.
Repent and believe the good news!"*   —Mark 1:15

Pastor Rick Warren says, "Repentance starts in the mind, not in actions. If you change your mind, your behavior will follow." Repentance actually starts with our minds making a U-turn. Repentance is turning away from ourselves, from sin, from lies, and toward God. When our eyes are solely fixed on Jesus, we're glad to leave the old, unprofitable ways behind. We press forward, eager to be like him in everything we do.

The opportunity for repentance is great news because it means that we are never stuck with who we are now. We're not stuck with a foggy brain, or with a habit of anxious thoughts, or with patterns of eating that drag us down. God offers us freedom and a fresh start, a clean slate no matter how many times we've needed one before. In Isaiah 30:15, God says, "In repentance and rest is your salvation."

If you're facing a time when repentance is necessary, look to Jesus and think about how excellent it will be to be more like him, to be closer to him, to feel his smile when he looks at you.

FOOD FOR THOUGHT

Seize the golden opportunity to make a U-turn and start fresh.

MORE AND MORE

And the Lord—who is the Spirit—makes us more and more like him as
we are changed into his glorious image.   *—2 Corinthians 3:18 NLT*

The Holy Spirit doesn't wave a magic wand and change your habits in a day. Your health habits and how you relate to people took decades to form, and the Spirit is going to change them over time if you cooperate with him. That's why Paul says the Spirit makes us *more and more* like the Lord over time, not all at once in one magic moment.

You can cooperate with him by embracing his tools of change: the Scriptures, prayer, and trusted friends who will hear the truth and tell you the truth. Spend daily time in the Word, and let the Spirit speak to you about your life. Spend weekly time with trusted friends who accept you for who you are. Little by little, more and more, you will see real change—not just in your health, but also in your resemblance to Christ. Small, steady steps will lead to big, lasting results in the end.

FOOD FOR THOUGHT

God is in the business of miracle makeovers.

TRUSTING OVER AND OVER

Trust in him at all times, you people; pour out your hearts to him, for God is our refuge. —Psalm 62:8

No matter how well we're doing with our health goals, we have good reason to go to God to pour out our hearts to him. Brennan Manning said, "My trust in God flows out of the experience of his loving me, day in and day out, whether the day is stormy or fair, whether I'm sick or in good health, whether I'm in a state of grace or disgrace. He comes to me where I live and loves me as I am."[3]

This is the great news: God loves us right where we are, and he's utterly patient with the progress we've made, no matter how small our steps look to us. He's like a good parent thrilled with the first steps of an infant. The child completely trusts the parent to hold him up when he wobbles. There is no doubt in his mind that his parent will respond with help and with delight. God is just like that.

FOOD FOR THOUGHT

God is our refuge, loving us as we are and comforting us when we need it.

DESIGNED FOR A BODY

*Then the LORD God formed a man from the dust of the ground and
breathed into his nostrils the breath of life, and the man became a living being.*
—Genesis 2:7

From the beginning of the world, you were designed to have a body. Your body wasn't an afterthought tacked on to your soul. The Bible says that when God formed the first human being, he made him from the physical stuff of the earth and breathed God's own Spirit or breath into him to make him a living being. Adam, the first man, was embodied from day one.

Treasure your body. God does. You are a wondrous body-mind-spirit person. He designed you to need plant food to nourish the cells of your body, water to hydrate those cells, exercise to make your muscles and internal organs work well. Needs aren't negative; he designed you to have them.

Instead of focusing on the aspects of your body that frustrate you, try celebrating what God made. Thank God for your body—your body is you.

FOOD FOR THOUGHT

Your body is a wondrous treasure designed by God himself.

PUTTING ON THE NEW SELF

You were taught, with regard to your former way of life, to put off your old self . . . to be made new in the attitude of your minds; and to put on the new self, created to be like God in true righteousness and holiness.

—Ephesians 4:22–24

Every time we have a thought, our brains release chemicals. When we have a sad, angry, anxious, hopeless, or helpless thought, our brains release chemicals that make us feel awful. Dr. Daniel Amen says negative thoughts make our hands colder, our muscle more tense, our breathing shallower, and our brainwaves disorganized.

When we have a happy, hopeful, encouraging, loving, or connected thought, our brains release a completely different set of chemicals. Our hands get warmer and drier, our muscles become more relaxed, and our breathing becomes slower and deeper.

Suppressing automatic negative thoughts doesn't work. Instead, we need to notice them, put words to them, and replace them with God's truth, such as a verse like Isaiah 41:10: "So do not fear, for I am with you. . . . I will strengthen you and help you."

Pay attention to the thoughts that go through your mind. Are negative or positive ones common? How do they affect you?

FOOD FOR THOUGHT

Refocusing your thoughts with truth will refresh your body and your soul.

ENERGY SOURCE

I am the vine; you are the branches. If you remain in me and I in you, you will bear much fruit; apart from me you can do nothing.

—*John 15:5*

God is the energy source behind all transformational change, and that includes getting healthy. He will not only show us the way, but will also give us the motivation and power to succeed as we look to him. Think how intimate the connection is between a grape vine and a branch. The branch has to be fully attached; otherwise, there's no flow of nutrients. That's how closely connected we need to be to Jesus, our vine.

We sometimes wonder why the change process is so up and down rather than smooth sailing. God doesn't tell us why, but this pattern does reinforce our dependence on him. If we sustain our connection to him through his Word and prayer, we find that our lives will bear the fruit of consistent and lasting change. As the psalmist said, "You make known to me the path of life; you will fill me with joy in your presence, with eternal pleasures at your right hand" (Psalm 16:11).

FOOD FOR THOUGHT

Cling to the vine to stay closely connected to the true source of life and joy.

QUESTION YOUR THOUGHTS

*You're blessed when you get your inside world—your mind and heart—
put right. Then you can see God in the outside world.*

—*Matthew 5:8 MSG*

I t's important not to believe every foolish thought that comes into our heads.

I'll never stay on this meal plan, it will be so hard!

This won't work for me.

Nothing I try works.

These negative thoughts predict a worst-case future. Yet if we act on these beliefs, then we will struggle and find ourselves with a self-fulfilling prophecy. Believing our negative thoughts can actually give us a negative outcome.

Research has shown that if we learn not to believe every foolish thing we think, it is helpful for weight loss. In a study in Sweden, where people were trained to talk back to their negative thoughts, they lost an average of seventeen pounds over ten weeks. Changing your thinking patterns has also been shown to be helpful in minimizing anxiety and panic attacks[4].

Write down your negative thoughts. Then ask yourself, "Is it true? How do I know?"

FOOD FOR THOUGHT

When you ditch worst-case thinking, you'll discover that hope and joy flow into your heart and mind.

A GENTLE WHISPER

The LORD was not in the fire. And after the fire came a gentle whisper.

—*1 Kings 19:12*

The prophet Elijah went to a remote place to meet with God. He was stretched to his limit and told God exactly how frustrated and discouraged he was. God sent a mighty windstorm, but God wasn't in the wind. Then God sent an earthquake, but God wasn't in the earthquake. Then God sent a fire, but God wasn't in the fire.

When God had Elijah's complete attention, God came to Elijah in a gentle whisper. God listened to Elijah, and God whispered gently but firmly what Elijah needed to hear.

God often speaks in a gentle whisper, so we need to silence the distractions—including the distractions inside our heads—in order to hear him. Consider turning off your phone, going to someplace quiet, and telling God what's on your mind. Then wait for his whisper. Even five or ten minutes in a busy day can make a big difference. Or if you're really at your limit, a day away with plenty of rest might make you more effective in the long run. He's waiting for you.

FOOD FOR THOUGHT

If you remove the distractions in your life, you'll hear God's gentle whisper.

ABUNDANT LIFE

I have come that they may have life, and have it to the full.

—*John 10:10*

The life God wants to give you is not small and restrictive. Jesus says the abundant life that comes from being intimately connected to him will be better than all your dreams rolled into one. It will happen more and more as you spend daily time with him. Create daily alerts in your phone or computer to remind you to check in with God. This will help you create a habit of spending time with him throughout the day. Just say, "Jesus, I'm here. I'm back. I trust in you."

Ask him to open your eyes to see his abundance through your work, in your health, and in your relationships. He wants to fill you with the abundance of his own life so that your life is rich and satisfying. He wants a real relationship with you, where you come to know him more deeply as time goes on. You'll find there's always more to learn. And you'll be amazed at how he surpasses your wildest dreams with the richness of his love and nearness of his presence.

FOOD FOR THOUGHT

Go ahead and dream of abundant life. God freely provides as we draw near to him.

FULFILLING YOUR CALLING

We constantly pray for you, that our God may make you worthy of his calling, and that by his power he may bring to fruition your every desire for goodness and your every deed prompted by faith.

—2 Thessalonians 1:11

The apostle Paul loved the believers in Thessalonica, and this is what he prayed for them. It is our prayer for you, too, and a good one to pray for yourself and others doing The Daniel Plan with you. Pray that God will fulfill every good purpose in your life. Pray that he will empower and make fruitful every action prompted by your faith as you become healthier and healthier for the glory of God.

Tell God you desire good fruit from your faith-inspired choices to practice The Daniel Plan. This isn't just a program you're doing because someone told you to do it. Let it be something that flows from your belief that God wants you full of life for years to come. Ask him to strengthen your body, mind, and spirit so that you live a life worthy of his calling. Not by sheer effort but by his grace.

FOOD FOR THOUGHT

Ask God to fulfill his good purposes in your life.

POWER IN WEAKNESS

But he said to me, "My grace is sufficient for you, for my power is made perfect in weakness." Therefore I will boast all the more gladly about my weaknesses, so that Christ's power may rest on me.

—2 Corinthians 12:9

Any process of change exposes our weaknesses. We want to make changes, but when we bump up against our weaknesses, we can get discouraged and think change is impossible. And it may be impossible—if we are on our own.

But we're not on our own. God has given us his free gift of the Holy Spirit who lives in us and empowers us. We only need to ask, "Holy Spirit, please help me to accomplish this," and he is there with us in power.

Don't expect him to make the process effortless or smooth, because he wants your weaknesses to show off the fact that his power is accomplishing everything. So don't demand perfection of yourself; aim for progress in little steps, and celebrate your weaknesses. When you are weak, God is strong. His grace truly is sufficient.

FOOD FOR THOUGHT

You can boast of your weaknesses when God is providing the power to overcome.

NOT EVERYTHING IS BENEFICIAL

"I have the right to do anything," you say—but not everything is beneficial.
"I have the right to do anything"—but I will not be mastered by anything.
—1 Corinthians 6:12

There are no forbidden foods, no foods that will defile us spiritually. However, while something may be permissible, it may not be beneficial. Some things aren't morally wrong, but they are unnecessary and unhealthy. They are not the best, most life-giving choice for us.

We don't want unwise choices to sneak in or begin to dominate our lives. We don't want to be mastered by sugar or anything else. If we find that some food or some habit has dominated us, such that we crave it if we don't have it, then we need to take charge of it and say no. God will give us the power to remove it from our lives if we ask him and keep asking. It may take time to uproot it from our lives, but we can become free of the things that aren't life-giving choices.

FOOD FOR THOUGHT

Sometimes pulling a few weeds in your life makes room for you to flourish the way God designed you.

WELLSPRING OF LIFE

And if the Spirit of him who raised Jesus from the dead is living in you, he who raised Christ from the dead will also give life to your mortal bodies because of his Spirit who lives in you. —Romans 8:11

The Holy Spirit lives in you. He is the Spirit who raised Jesus' body from the dead. God promises that he will also give life to your mortal body. His presence in you is one reason your body is of immense value. He offers you new life, strength, comfort, and hope to move forward in the way God designed you.

Ask him today to fulfill that promise. The ultimate fulfillment will come when he raises you from the dead and gives you a glorified body for all eternity. But eternal life starts now, and you can invite the Spirit to give life to your body now. What do you need strength for today? What hope do you need to overcome discouragement? Reach out to God in faith, asking him to fill you with his Spirit.

FOOD FOR THOUGHT

The Spirit who raised Jesus from the dead lives in you. Imagine the new life he desires to give you by the working of his Spirit in you.

BOUGHT AT A PRICE

You are not your own; you were bought at a price. Therefore honor God with your bodies. —1 Corinthians 6:19–20

God made your body and gave it to you. As Psalm 139:13 says, "you knit me together in my mother's womb." He then bought you out of slavery to sin at the price of Jesus' shed blood on the cross. He bought all of you: body, soul, and spirit. So he is the owner of your body, and you are the manager of it, caring for it and putting it to work on his behalf. Your body is a priceless gift on loan to you, to be used for his glory.

Therefore, God calls you to treat your body with respect. It is holy to God, and he trusts you to care for it. What do you plan to do with your body today? What will you feed it? How will you care for it so that it works well for many years? What exercise does it need? How much sleep? What work would honor him?

FOOD FOR THOUGHT

Your body is a tremendous gift that God lends to you so that you can use it for his glory.

GIVE ME UNDERSTANDING

Your hands made me and formed me; give me understanding to learn your
commands. —Psalm 119:73

Who knows better than God what is going to make you healthy? He made your body and set in motion the laws by which it functions. The Bible says, "Give me the sense to follow your commands" (Psalm 119:73 NLT). We need to understand the laws by which our bodies work, and we also need to have the good sense to follow them.

Deuteronomy 32:47 says God's laws aren't just idle words. They are the source of our very life. By obeying them, we will have long life in the land where God puts us. This is true of the natural laws God wove into our bodies, just as it's true of the laws written down in the Bible. Nobody gets exempted from the laws of nature.

Pray to understand the kind of fuel your body needs in order to be fully nourished. Pray to understand and heed your body's need for fellowship, exercise, and rest. If you ask, he will give you the understanding and the strength to follow his laws.

FOOD FOR THOUGHT

God longs to give you the understanding to heed his commands.

ENDURING FAITH

When your faith is tested, your endurance has a chance to grow. So let it grow, for when your endurance is fully developed, you will be perfect and complete.   —James 1:3–4 NLT

Charles Spurgeon said, "No faith is so precious as that which lives and triumphs in adversity. Tried faith brings experience. You could not have believed your own weakness had you not been compelled to pass through the rivers; and you would never have known God's strength had you not been supported amid the floods."[5]

Each time we experience our weakness in a trial, we can thank God for showing us our weakness. And each time God's strength carries us through, we can thank him for his strength and for how our endurance will grow. Faith that goes through trials is like gold refined by fire; it reveals what is precious and beautiful. God wants us to learn endurance, and the only way to learn it is to endure, day after day.

FOOD FOR THOUGHT

Adversity can build our endurance. God is our coach, cheering us on and enabling us to do what we couldn't do on our own.

TALKING BACK

I've already run for dear life straight to the arms of God.

—*Psalm 11:1 MSG*

Suppose you have a bad day and you think, *I can't do this program anymore. I'm not strong enough, I'm not confident enough, I've had too many failures, I just ate a double-double cheeseburger and then I went for the ice cream after that, because I'm feeling overwhelmed.*

The important thing to do in that moment is to run straight to God. Tell him exactly how you feel and what you think. Confess the thoughts that are plaguing you, and ask him to renew your mind. With God's help, reframe those thoughts with truth.

"I had a bad day today, but I got good information from it. I learned that I sometimes make unhealthy food choices when I feel overwhelmed. God, please help me lean on you and others for support in my life."

Do you see how this positive outlook is a deeper truth than what you believed before you went to God? Deliberately choose to rehearse this new perspective in your mind. And stay in God's presence where truth and peace reign.

FOOD FOR THOUGHT

On bad days, run straight into the arms of God and let his truth change your perspective.

THE SECRET OF LONG LIFE

Do not forget my teaching, but keep my commands in your heart, for they will prolong your life many years and bring you peace and prosperity.
—*Proverbs 3:1–2*

Many people want to know the secret of prolonged life, peace, and prosperity. Here it is: obeying God. If we keep his commands, we can expect a much longer life than if we ignore them. These commands referred to in Proverbs include the range of choices that the Bible calls wisdom, the practical understanding of how to live well.

Loving our neighbors is wisdom. Doing an appropriate amount of work—without laziness but with enough rest—is wisdom. Caring for our bodies is wisdom. Worshiping the Lord and rejecting all lesser gods is wisdom. Getting rid of destructive habits is wisdom.

What is God asking of you today? Is he calling you to reach out to someone in love? Is he asking you to give up a destructive habit? Is he asking you to take a step to care for your body? Whatever it is, if you follow his commands, they will lead you down the road to peace and life.

FOOD FOR THOUGHT

Peace and wholeness come from taking the Lord's commands to heart.

LEAN NOT ON YOUR UNDERSTANDING

Trust in the LORD with all your heart and lean not on your own understanding; in all your ways submit to him, and he will make your paths straight. —*Proverbs 3:5–6*

If you feel that your understanding isn't up to the task of absorbing the available information about your health, there's good news: you shouldn't depend on your own understanding anyway. Learn what you can, and, even more importantly, trust the Lord to guide you. Submit your eating habits, your daily movement, and everything else to him, and he will make your paths straight. Pray for guidance. Ask him what your next steps should be.

This doesn't mean you shouldn't try to understand what to eat or how to exercise. It means you don't need to stress over it. It also means it's unwise to assume that you know it all already. Open your mind and heart to new information that God wants to give you. Allow him to guide you to take steps toward health. How will you trust the Lord today?

FOOD FOR THOUGHT

You can entrust everything to the Lord; he longs to make your paths straight.

ENVY

A heart at peace gives life to the body, but envy rots the bones.

—Proverbs 14:30

It's not just what you eat that counts, but what is eating you. "Envy" happens when someone else has something good, and you either desire to have it, desire them to lose it, or constantly compare your life to theirs. Envy is one of the most corrosive attitudes you can allow into your heart. Envy grows when you are blind to the good things God has given you, or when you are ungrateful for them, and instead focus on what everyone else seems to have. It robs you of peace and causes stress.

The antidote for envy is gratitude (Psalm 100:4). Look at the good things you have and thank God for them. Don't think of yourself as deprived and the other person as undeservedly gifted. If you tend to think of yourself as deprived, stop and question that thought. Has God really not given you what you need to flourish? No, he has given you everything you need for life and godliness (2 Peter 1:3).

FOOD FOR THOUGHT

Set your heart at peace by replacing envious thoughts with grateful ones. Enter God's gates with thanksgiving.

THE FREEDOM OF CONFESSION

When I kept silent, my bones wasted away through my groaning all day long. . . . my strength was sapped as in the heat of summer.

—Psalm 32:3–4

Confessing sin is good for your health. God didn't design us to carry guilt and resentment in our hearts. In Psalm 32, David says that when he refused to confess his sins, he was weak and miserable. His strength evaporated. When he finally stopped hiding his sins from God and confessed them, God forgave them and his guilt was gone. Even his body felt better with that weight off his mind. He ends Psalm 32 with a shout of joy.

If there is anything on your conscience right now, why not confess it to God and let it go? It might also help you to confess it to one trusted person who won't judge you, who will keep what you say private, and who will encourage you to stay on the right path. Nothing is healthier for you than a clear conscience—and knowing your sins are forgiven.

FOOD FOR THOUGHT

Confession is good for the soul and for the body.

THE SOURCE OF MOTIVATION

My counsel is this: Live freely, animated and motivated by God's Spirit.
Then you won't feed the compulsions of selfishness.

—*Galatians 5:16 MSG*

Did you know that God gives you the motivation to do what he wants you to do? This includes the motivation to get physically healthy. He gives you not just the power to do it, but also the desire to do it. The motivation to do God's will actually comes from God himself.

So if you don't already desire to get physically healthy so much that you're willing to schedule movement into your calendar or take healthy steps with your eating, ask God to give you that desire. If you aren't motivated to get enough rest or take time alone with God each day, ask him for the motivation. Tell him, "Lord, I don't want to make these healthy changes, but I *want* to want to make them. It's been tough trying to shift my mindset, but I desire to do that. Please fill me with your Holy Spirit, so that I love what you promise and desire what you command." He longs to answer that prayer.

FOOD FOR THOUGHT

God is eager to give you the motivation to make the healthy changes you desire.

TRUE NOURISHMENT

Do not be wise in your own eyes; fear the LORD and shun evil. This will bring health to your body and nourishment to your bones.

—*Proverbs 3:7–8*

This proverb invites you to "fear the Lord"—take him and his commands seriously, have more concern for what he thinks than for what anybody else thinks, put his opinion way ahead of your opinion. Fearing the Lord will lead you to run like crazy away from evil behavior and toward his loving embrace.

Why does fearing the Lord lead to health? Because the Lord knows what is good for your body and soul. He made them, so he has the wisdom to guide you in how to take care of them. If you are teachable, he will teach you. He promises to guide you on the path he desires.

One of the great things about fearing the Lord is that it drives out all other fears. When you know that pleasing the Lord is your number one priority, then other fears dwindle and fall away.

FOOD FOR THOUGHT

Tranquility and true nourishment come from trusting the Lord and letting him direct your path.

GOD IS LOVE

*No one has ever seen God; but if we love one another, God lives in us and
his love is made complete in us.*   —1 John 4:12

If we want lasting change, we must fill our lives with love. Why?
Because love can change the unchangeable. Love is the most powerful force in the universe, because "God is love" (1 John 4:8).

John doesn't say God has love; he says God *is* love. Love is the
essence of what God is. God is Father, Son, and Spirit in an eternal
relationship of love.

Love invigorates. Love revitalizes. Love renews. Love refreshes.
Love heals. Love strengthens. Love gives you energy when you don't
have energy. Love empowers you when you don't have the power.
We need God's kind of love if we are going to fulfill the purposes for
which we were made.

So as you seek lasting change today, invite God's love to touch
those areas of your life that need healing in a deeper way. Then look
for opportunities to give that love away to others.

FOOD FOR THOUGHT

God's love can change the unchangeable so that we
are able to love others with the love we've received.
What a privilege!

FINDING THE COURAGE TO CHANGE

Be strong and courageous.

—*Joshua 1:6*

Have you ever read this verse and tried to be stronger and more courageous? The key to deep and lasting change isn't trying harder. Pastor Rick Warren says, "God specializes in miracle makeovers." Try to imagine what good changes could happen in your life if you depended on God's infinite power instead of your own willpower.

Effort is necessary, but it's effort fueled by the power of God's Holy Spirit. The Bible says, "Be energetic in your life of salvation, reverent and sensitive before God. That energy is *God's* energy, an energy deep within you, God himself willing and working at what will give him the most pleasure" (Philippians 2:12–13 MSG).

God loves you so much that he freely puts his power to work in your life. He wants to be the one who is shown to be victorious. That's why he works so powerfully in the lives of weak and humble people. For what do you need his power today?

FOOD FOR THOUGHT

Bring all of your weaknesses to God and receive from him the power to be strong and courageous.

GOD'S DWELLING PLACE

Do you not know that your bodies are temples of the Holy Spirit, who is in you, whom you have received from God? —1 Corinthians 6:19

In the Old Testament, God dwelt in the holiest part of the temple. Only the high priest was allowed to go there, and only once a year (Leviticus 16:2; Hebrews 9:7). Anyone who violated that law died. That's how holy the presence of God is in his temple.

But now, since God has raised Jesus from the dead and sent his Spirit to his people, your mortal body is a temple of that Holy Spirit. Your body is like the holiest part of the Old Testament temple. It is a sacred place. It matters to God.

Put your hand on your chest, close your eyes, and sit with the idea that the Holy Spirit dwells there now. Pray that God will allow you to fully embrace your body as his temple, so that you can honor it as a sacred place in all you do.

FOOD FOR THOUGHT

You are a temple where God's Holy Spirit has taken up residence. You are sacred space!

THURSDAY

HIS GLORIOUS RICHES

*I pray that out of his glorious riches he may strengthen you with power
through his Spirit in your inner being.* —Ephesians 3:16

God has glorious, unlimited resources to offer you. Out of those glorious riches, he will give you mighty inner strength through his Holy Spirit. And he's never going to get tired of helping you. He never gives up. He never gets frustrated. He's strong even when you stumble. If you fall down, he'll pick you up. If you get off the path, he'll show where to U-turn and guide you back on to his straight path.

How does that happen? It happens as you come to God and make your declaration of *dependence*. You're not independent; you're dependent on him for everything. Ask him daily—even hourly—to give you the strength to do his will in his way for his glory. Don't try to go it alone one more day.

FOOD FOR THOUGHT

God longs to give you the strength to do his will in his way for his glory.

AN INCREDIBLE PARTNERSHIP

Commit to the LORD whatever you do, and he will establish your plans.
—Proverbs 16:3

How can your plan for healthiness and balance succeed? You need two things: prayer and diligence. Prayer and diligence are like two sides of the same coin. You pray as if it all depends on God, and you work as if it all depends on you. Putting your whole effort into something feels so different when you have prayed about it and God is empowering you in it.

Committing to the Lord whatever you do means saying, "God, I'm committing to you another day, one day at a time. I want to be healthier at the end of the day than I was when I got up this morning. Please give me the strength to do my part in that." That's the pray part. Proverbs 13:4 says, "The desires of the diligent are fully satisfied." In other words, you've got to work. It takes faith, food, fitness, focus, and friends. You eat right; you exercise. You focus your thoughts on Scripture. You get enough sleep. You build community. That's the diligence part.

FOOD FOR THOUGHT

Transformation is super-powered when you are diligent, devoted, and dependent.

THE SECRET SAUCE

Plans fail for lack of counsel, but with many advisers they succeed.

—Proverbs 15:22

When we talk over our plans with other people and get their input, we are far more likely to succeed. Who are your advisers? They should be people you connect with regularly. Perhaps those who are partnering with you in The Daniel Plan, your small group, or your spouse. Whoever they are, for a few minutes each day or week, encourage each other, challenge each other, share the joy of successes or the sadness of sorrow, discuss questions or concerns. Ride the ups and downs together.

It's a good idea to have more than one adviser. Then you will be able to benefit from a diversity of perspectives. You may have one or two people who are closest to you but then draw on the wisdom of a wider circle for specific areas of your life.

These people will help you keep moving forward. This is how people find lasting change—when they share the journey. If you haven't asked someone to partner with you yet, go for it. It will be a blessing to them too.

FOOD FOR THOUGHT

Friends are the secret ingredients that will make your plans flourish.

GOD'S PATIENCE

The Lord is not slow in keeping his promise, as some understand slowness. Instead he is patient with you, not wanting anyone to perish, but everyone to come to repentance. —2 Peter 3:9

God is patient. Almost 2,000 years have passed since Christ's resurrection, and still he postpones Christ's return to judge the world. He wants to give as many people as possible time to repent and turn to him.

If God is patient with all of humankind to that degree, even with people who don't believe he exists, he is certainly patient with us who do believe in him. If it takes time and numerous setbacks for us to become spiritually mature, he is neither surprised nor frustrated. The Bible tells us nine times that he is slow to anger (Psalm 86:15).

God is proud of us for running the race he has set before us. He who began a good work in us will carry it on to completion (Philippians 1:6). He has plenty of time.

FOOD FOR THOUGHT

No matter how long growth takes us, God has infinite patience with us. He keeps providing his power and grace all the way to the finish line.

ETERNAL MOTIVATION

May our Lord Jesus Christ himself and God our Father, who loved us and by his grace gave us eternal encouragement and good hope, encourage your hearts and strengthen you in every good deed and word.

—*2 Thessalonians 2:16–17*

When we are pursuing healthy changes, there's nothing we need more than eternal encouragement and good hope. That's motivation. We need to be strengthened in every good deed and word, because we can't be transformed by willpower alone.

God will often work through people. Who offers you encouragement when you need it? They are gifts from God. How can you spend more time with those people or welcome their help more often? Soak up their support, and thank them for their role in your life.

God's Word is another essential source of encouragement. Consider committing to memory a verse that fills you with encouragement and strength.

Through other people and his Word, God will provide the encouragement and strength you need to reach your goals.

FOOD FOR THOUGHT

Encouragement and hope will motivate you to keep going even when it's difficult. These are priceless treasures that God wants to lavish on you.

MOVEMENT YOU ENJOY

He gives strength to the weary and increases the power of the weak.
—*Isaiah 40:29*

When we were young, moving our bodies was a natural part of every day. We looked forward to recess. We called it "play," and we loved every minute of it. Now we often call it "exercise" and avoid it. So the key to recovering the joy of movement is to find ways to integrate fun, laughter, devotion, and adventure into all aspects of movement. We can lift our arms over our heads and praise God for giving strength to the weary and increasing the power of the weak. We can use stretching breaks to remind us to let go of control and cast our anxieties onto God (1 Peter 5:7). We can experiment with playful aerobic activities that may actually bring smiles to our faces.

God wants us to enjoy moving our bodies. He made them to move. What forms of movement would be fun for you if you were confident that God would give you strength and increase your power?

FOOD FOR THOUGHT

Physical movement is meant to include joy and devotion.

SPURRING ONE ANOTHER ON

Let us consider how we may spur one another on toward love and good deeds.
—*Hebrews 10:24*

Spurring one another on means being willing to help others become all that God desires and reminding them of what is true about their new identities—even when they can't see it at all themselves. It means helping them to stand up when they fall—with no condemnation—and setting a gracious pace for them when it's hard for them to keep going.

How would you like to be stirred up to love and good deeds? Think about a time when someone else encouraged you in a way that boosted your confidence or motivation. Then do that very same thing for someone else.

We can also partner with others by inviting them to join us in how God is asking us to live: "Come along with me. I can't do this on my own. We would be better together." The habit of encouragement is often more easily caught than taught.

FOOD FOR THOUGHT

If you want to be spurred on to love, try spurring on someone else who needs encouragement from you.

ULTIMATE HOPE

We do not want you to be uninformed about those who sleep in death, so that you do not grieve like the rest of mankind, who have no hope.
—*1 Thessalonians 4:13*

Billy Graham said, "The Bible says that as Christians we don't grieve the same way people do who have no hope of eternity and of Heaven—but we still grieve."[6] We know we'll see our loved ones again in heaven, but we are still sad when they leave this earthly life.

Part of grief is accepting our feelings about any loss, whether the loss of health or a job or a relationship. Every loss is real and deserves to be grieved.

We need to know how to grieve so that losses don't drive us to make unhealthy choices to numb our pain. We need to feel the pain and welcome the support of others, so that over time we can move through the loss and find comfort in Christ.

FOOD FOR THOUGHT

One day God will wipe every tear from our eyes (Revelation 21:4) and grief will be only a memory.

THE BIG DIFFERENCE

I do not understand what I do. For what I want to do I do not do, but what I hate I do. —Romans 7:15

Have you experienced this pattern when you tried to make healthy changes? You can't always make yourself do right. You want to, but you can't. And when you try not to do the wrong thing, you do it anyway. Why does this happen?

We all have an old nature with deeply rooted habits inside us. It loves to do those wrong things that have become routine for us. We can't break free of those habits on our own, and the apostle Paul went on to write, "Who will free me from slavery to this deadly lower nature?" Then he gives the answer, "Thank God, Christ Jesus has done it. He has set me free."

In Romans 7, Paul uses the words "I, me, my" twenty-seven times. But in Romans 8 he uses the word "Spirit" nineteen times. That's the difference between defeat and victory: trusting in "me" versus surrendering to the Holy Spirit.

FOOD FOR THOUGHT

God's Spirit is ready and waiting to break you free of old patterns and move a new direction.

SATURDAY

NO CONDEMNATION

There is now no condemnation for those who are in Christ Jesus.

—*Romans 8:1*

All change starts with acceptance. Until you feel accepted by God, you're going to continue to be caught in a cycle of defeat, failure, guilt, and recrimination. The greatest chapter on change in Scripture begins by saying, if you belong to Christ, God does not condemn you. Are you everything you need to be? No. Are you in the best shape you could be? No. But God says, "There is no condemnation." He welcomes you to a path not of perfection, but of ongoing change.

Instead of being motivated about these changes out of guilt, pressure, or fear of not measuring up, let God's acceptance encourage you. Your worthiness comes from your relationship to Christ because you're forgiven. You're cleansed. The Holy Spirit has freed you from the vicious cycle of sin and death. You're living by grace, not by condemnation.

FOOD FOR THOUGHT

If you struggle today, remind yourself that there is no condemnation for you, but rather God's full acceptance and welcome.

MASTERED BY THE MASTER

For the Spirit God gave us does not make us timid, but gives us power, love and self-discipline. —2 Timothy 1:7

God promises to give you the power to remain faithful to the commitments you make. God doesn't give you a spirit of fear or shyness. Feeling overwhelmed by what it will take to get healthy is not from him. He's not giving you insecurity or worry or anxiety. He gives you power, love, and self-discipline.

Did you know that true self-discipline comes from God? Self-control actually comes from giving control to God. The more you surrender to him and give up control of your life, the more self-control you have. When you're mastered by the Master, you are mastered by nothing else. But if he's not your Master in practical daily ways, anything can master your life.

Where in your life are you struggling with self-discipline? Instead of doubling down on yourself, yield that area to God. Make it a daily offering to him.

FOOD FOR THOUGHT

Self-control comes from giving control to God. That's true freedom from fear, cravings, and anything else that burdens you.

APPRECIATING YOUR BODY

Has not the one God made you? You belong to him in body and spirit.

—*Malachi 2:15*

D r. Mark Hyman says, "What you put on your fork dictates whether you are sick or well, slim or fat, depleted or energized. Real food has the power to give you your life back so you can more fully engage in the purpose for your life." If real food has this power, you can be sure that God cares what you eat. He wants you to appreciate and give dignity to your body by nourishing it the way he designed it to be nourished.

What motivates you to appreciate your body? Maybe the very idea of appreciating it is new for you. If so, stop and think about it. Can you name five things you appreciate about your body? Here are three: God made it, Jesus died for it, and the Holy Spirit dwells in it. There are many more. Think of how wondrously it works, the many ways it moves, and what it enables you to do.

FOOD FOR THOUGHT

Your body is an amazing creation, crafted to give glory to the one who made it.

LIFE AND PEACE

The mind governed by the flesh is death, but the mind governed by the
Spirit is life and peace.   —Romans 8:6

Every time we try to do something on our own, we're going to hit a
brick wall, but every time we let God's Spirit work in and through
us, we're going to find life and peace. Our goal in The Daniel Plan is
not that we look better. Our goal is not even that we just have more
energy. Our goal is to experience life in its fullness, the life the Holy
Spirit wants to give us.

The Daniel Plan starts the pursuit of full life at the fundamental
level of our bodies. Why? Because everything God wants to do in us,
through us, to us, and for us, he wants to do in our bodies. If our bodies aren't healthy enough, how can we serve him? We need our bodies
to pray, proclaim the gospel, and help the needy. So we're after God-
empowered change in our whole lives.

FOOD FOR THOUGHT

Abundant life and peace is meant for your soul and
your body.

CONFIDENT EXPECTATIONS

We were given this hope when we were saved. (If we already have something, we don't need to hope for it. But if we look forward to something we don't yet have, we must wait patiently and confidently.)
—Romans 8:24–25 NLT

We are saved by trusting God. Trusting means looking forward to getting something we don't yet have. A person who already has something doesn't need to hope and trust that he'll get it. But if we must keep trusting God for something that hasn't happened yet, the delay teaches us to wait patiently and confidently.

Biblical hope isn't just a wish. It's a confident expectation. We are confident that what God has promised for us on earth and for eternity, he will fulfill. We are so confident that we can even thank him in advance for what he has promised to do. We might pray, "God, thank you for The Daniel Plan. Thank you that, with your strength, it's going to be different this time. Thank you that I have no condemnation, that I have your Spirit, and that I can trust in you. No matter how much time this takes, I am waiting with confident hope in you."

FOOD FOR THOUGHT

God's promises are certain; we can thank him in advance for everything he has promised.

ALL THINGS WORK TOGETHER

And we know that in all things God works for the good of those who love him, who have been called according to his purpose.

—Romans 8:28

In all things, all that happens to us, God is working for our good if we love him and are conforming our lives to his plans. God says he will work it all for good.—even the relapses, even the failures, even the mistakes, even the setbacks. God says, "You know what? I'll fit that into the plan too. I will do it all for good if you will trust me."

Maybe you've had one failure after another in your attempts to live a healthier life. That's okay. God can even use that.

Maybe you are genetically inclined to a certain difficulty, or you grew up in a family that had many challenges. God can use even these things for good in your life if you give him all the pieces. What is in your life that you doubt God can turn to good?

FOOD FOR THOUGHT

Give God all the ups and downs you're dealing with; he promises to use them for good.

GOD LASTS

Why would you ever complain, O Jacob . . . , saying, "GOD has lost track of me. He doesn't care what happens to me"? . . . GOD doesn't come and go. God lasts. He's Creator of all you can see or imagine. He doesn't get tired out, doesn't pause to catch his breath. And he knows everything, inside and out.
—Isaiah 40:27–28 MSG

In the challenges of life, do you ever feel like God has lost track of you? We may feel lost, but he doesn't come and go. He lasts. He rides through the ups and the downs with us. We may get tired, but he never does. When we're weary, we can lean on him, because he never loses patience with us. No matter how many down days we have, God is always ready to start fresh.

He also knows everything, inside and out. If you aren't sure what to aim at, ask him to show you. When it comes to your health, you can ask him what he desires for you, what are your next steps, and he'll be right there with an answer. He desires to use your life; his vision goes beyond the limitations of what you can see.

FOOD FOR THOUGHT

God cares intimately about all that happens to you, and he has a unique vision of who you can become.

THE CHEERFUL HEART

The cheerful heart has a continual feast.

—Proverbs 15:15

The circumstances of our lives can be up or down, but a cheerful heart isn't at the mercy of circumstances. If we are able to take a step back and deliberately bring our attention to the things that are going right in our lives, the blessings we have, we can find something to rejoice in. During certain seasons filled with hardship, we may have to look hard for the blessings, but they are there. We don't pretend that the cancer or the financial struggle isn't happening, but we choose gratefulness for the blessings that are also there: for friendships or family or home or the constant presence of a loving God.

A popular saying is that life is 10 percent what happens to us and 90 percent how we react to it. So we have a choice to react by focusing on what we can be thankful for. Even if it's difficult, Proverbs 17:22 says a cheerful heart is good medicine.

"Where you bring your attention determines how you feel," Dr. Daniel Amen says, "and feeling grateful is a joyous place to be."

FOOD FOR THOUGHT

If we choose cheerfulness as our dominant outlook on life, our body and soul will benefit.

GOD IS FOR US

What, then, shall we say ... If God is for us, who can be against us?

—Romans 8:31

God did not spare his own Son from death, but gave him up for us. Doesn't that show that he's pulling for us?

God is for you. He wants you to succeed. He wants you to have more energy so that you can serve and glorify him, not just with your spirit, but also with your mind and body.

You are on God's team, and he is rooting for you as you step up to bat. As you depend on him, he will do everything in his unlimited power to enable you to become what he formed you to be. He's on your side. So if anybody else is against you, it doesn't matter. They don't count compared to God. If a voice inside your head tears you down, stop listening to it. Instead, hear God's truth about you: "Who then is the one who condemns? No one. Christ Jesus who died—more than that, who was raised to life—is at the right hand of God and is also interceding for us" (Romans 8:34). Count on that.

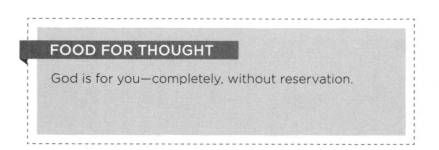

FOOD FOR THOUGHT

God is for you—completely, without reservation.

THE MOST OF EVERY OPPORTUNITY

Make the most of every opportunity. The days are evil.
                                    —*Ephesians 5:16 NIrV*

To make the most of every opportunity, it's good to make a plan. A plan clarifies what's important in your life. When you have a plan with goals, you then calculate how much time it's going to take to reach those goals—how much time weekly for how many weeks. But until it gets on your calendar, it's just a dream. You will find it much clearer in your mind and much more likely to happen if you write it all down.

One more step that will make an enormous difference in whether you follow through with your plan is telling somebody about your goal. Did you know that when you share your goal with somebody else, and commit to reporting back to that person, you have a 95 percent chance of achieving it?

What is your goal? What time on what days of the week are you going to give to it?

FOOD FOR THOUGHT

Take advantage of the opportunities before you.

WHAT IT TAKES TO GROW

Catch for us the foxes, the little foxes that ruin the vineyards.
—Song of Solomon 2:15

Be ruthless with distractions. They are like foxes let loose in a vineyard. They will eat the fruit and dig up the roots if you don't get rid of them.

Another way to think of distractions is like peach farming. When a peach tree blooms, it has a hundred little peaches on every branch. They will all grow to be smaller than golf balls. You have to pull off two-thirds of them and throw them away when they're tiny so that the tree can put its energy into growing thirty big peaches on each branch instead of a hundred tiny ones.

Like the peach tree, you will bear better fruit if you concentrate your energy. What are the few important things you need to do in your day? What are the distractions you need to ruthlessly eliminate? They may be good things, but if they're not important enough, you'll benefit from letting them go.

FOOD FOR THOUGHT

If you're ruthless about the distractions, you'll flourish in the areas God has planned for you.

A STEADFAST MIND

You will keep in perfect peace those whose minds are steadfast, because they trust in you.
—*Isaiah 26:3*

Asteadfast mind is crucial, because whatever gets your attention gets you. Your life will flourish if you simply stop focusing on what you *don't* want and start focusing on what you *do* want. Stop focusing on what's bad for you, and start focusing on what's good for you. Stop focusing on what everybody else wants you to do, and start focusing on what God wants you to do.

No matter what handicap you have, you can be healthier than you are right now. But there are choices to make. Choose to do things that will increase your energy. Choose things that will lower your stress and bring more power and more health in your life. Eat better, get more sleep, and prioritize what's important. Be steadfast about every choice and trust God for the results.

FOOD FOR THOUGHT

You'll find peace when you are steadfast about your choices and your focus.

BETTER TOGETHER

Two are better than one, because they have a good return for their labor....
A cord of three strands is not quickly broken.   —*Ecclesiastes 4:9, 12*

Friends are the "secret sauce" in The Daniel Plan. We make and sustain change so much better together. Our research in the first year of the program showed that people lost almost twice as much weight doing The Daniel Plan in a group rather than alone. Groups maximized people's ability to make desired improvements to their health.

Poor health habits are a community problem, so they need a community cure. Dr. Daniel Amen says health habits are contagious. If you spend time with people who exercise and eat healthily, you will be more likely to exercise and eat in a healthy way. Family and friends are key. Exercise is more fun with a buddy. Even negative thought patterns are easier to overcome with friends who can reinforce the positives. Don't try to go it alone; do your best to find at least one person to partner with you in the process toward better health.

FOOD FOR THOUGHT

If you want to sustain a healthy lifestyle, friends are invaluable.

METAMORPHOSIS

*And ... put on the new self, which is being renewed in knowledge in the
image of its Creator.* —Colossians 3:10

Change is always a choice. Nobody can force you or talk you into change. You will not change until you decide you actually want to.

Yet change is also wholly dependent on God. We can't become the flourishing, loving creatures we were made to be by sheer effort alone. We choose to change, and God gives us the power to change. Then gradually, over time, we do change, putting on the new self that God envisioned for us before the world was created.

Do you know what the word *transformation* is in Greek? It's the Greek word *metamorphosis*. Scientists use this word to describe the way a tadpole—a creature that can live only in the water—changes into a frog that can breathe on land. Putting on the new self is as radical as growing lungs that can breathe the rich, clean air of God's realm.

Let God transform you into a new person by changing the way you think. Let him give you the motivation to change.

FOOD FOR THOUGHT

God is ready to transform you into the image of your Creator.

HANGING OUT ON GOD'S PATH

We're in no hurry, GOD. We're content to linger in the path sign-posted with your decisions. Who you are and what you've done are all we'll ever want.
—Isaiah 26:8 MSG

Most of us are wasting first-class energy on second-class causes. We don't know the difference between what's urgent and what's important. The urgent is rarely the most important thing. In fact, what's most important in your life is often the easiest to set aside.

For instance, we want to spend time with God, but we set it aside for what's urgent. We want to spend time with our families, but we set it aside for what's urgent. The urgent often pushes the important out of the way. Yet a lot of things that seem urgent today aren't going to matter tomorrow.

The secret to an unhurried but productive life is focus. Is it productive to try to do fifty things that you dabble in? Probably not. What are the top five important things in your life that God has laid out for you specifically? If you know what's most important to God and do those few things, you don't need to worry about anything else.

FOOD FOR THOUGHT

Spend first-class energy on the things that are truly important.

FAITH OR FEAR?

"According to your faith let it be done to you."

—*Matthew 9:29*

Charles Stanley said, "Basically, there are two paths you can walk: faith or fear."[9] Faith is the confidence that God is helping you every step of the way on his plan for your life. It's the conviction that God is good, no matter what challenges or setbacks come your way. It consistently moves toward God with your needs.

How are you expecting God to help you on your journey toward better health? Faith is expecting God to fulfill his promises and help you do what he has called you to do. It is the difference between thinking, *God* might *help me get healthier* and *God* will *help me get healthier*.

The Bible says, "Let us draw near to God with a sincere heart and with the full assurance that faith brings" (Hebrews 10:22). Do you have that full assurance? It's not some psychological state that you try to conjure up in yourself. It comes as you meditate on God's promises and let them sink deeply into your heart.

FOOD FOR THOUGHT

If our hearts are turned toward God in faith, we can be confident that he will help us redesign our lives.

A DREAM WITH A DEADLINE

*One thing I do: Forgetting what is behind and straining toward what is
ahead, I press on toward the goal to win the prize for which God has called
me heavenward in Christ Jesus.* —Philippians 3:13–14

Long-term goals keep you from being discouraged by short-term
setbacks. Everybody has setbacks. Most of us have them every
day. But if you have a long-term goal and you're focused on it, then
short-term setbacks don't slow you down.

A goal is a dream with a deadline. A goal says, "By the end of this
year, I'm going to have this job, I'm going to weigh this amount, I'm
going to have read this number of books . . ." It's specific; it's measurable; it's timely.

What is your dream? What has God put on your heart? Spend
some time reflecting, as long as it takes, to put words to your dream.
Then give it a realistic deadline. Don't make it "someday;" give it a
date. Then you can ask God for the wisdom and steps to reach that
deadline. Remember, this isn't a dream you can fulfill on your own;
it's something God wants to fulfill.

FOOD FOR THOUGHT

Turn your dreams into goals, and let God help you
fulfill them.

ONE ANOTHER

Encourage one another daily, as long as it is called "Today."
—*Hebrews 3:13*

The phrase "one another" is used fifty-eight times in the New Testament. It says love one another, care for one another, encourage one another, support one another, pray for one another, greet one another, and share with one another.

The word *support* carries the idea of strengthening one another. Help one another become more capable of facing the challenges of health and living for Christ.

So reach out for support, and also consider who needs support from you today. Biblical fellowship is a radical level of friendship and community that implies deep commitment out of genuine and joyful love for one another.

God wired us in such a way that we need each other. We get well in community. You need your coworkers, your family, the people who sit near you in church, the parents of your children's friends—even if you don't yet know their names, or even if you find them difficult at times.

FOOD FOR THOUGHT

With a loving community of friends, you'll be better able to cope with challenges like fatigue, fear, frustration, failure, depression, and despair. And most importantly, you won't have to walk through them alone.

WHAT LIFE IS ABOUT

"Love the Lord your God with all your heart and with all your soul and with all your mind. . . . Love your neighbor as yourself."

—Matthew 22:37, 39

One day Jesus was walking down the street, and a man came up and asked, "Lord, what's life all about?"

Jesus told him life is all about love. It's not about accomplishment. It's not about acquisition. It's not about popularity, power, or prestige. It's about love. It's about relationships. You can summarize all of life in two phrases: love God with all your heart, and love your neighbor as yourself. This is called the Great Commandment: make the connection with God, and make the connection with others. If you don't have those two loves, then you miss the purpose of life.

Sometimes we get wrapped up in urgent things that have nothing to do with love. By contrast, our goal in The Daniel Plan is to build our lives on a foundation of love. As Mother Teresa said, "Do ordinary things with extraordinary love."[10] How can you reach out in love today?

FOOD FOR THOUGHT

If you focus on love, you'll live a full life and influence others for Christ far beyond your expectations.

THE LORD'S SERVANT

"I am the Lord's servant," Mary answered. *"May your word to me be
fulfilled."* —Luke 1:38

Mary received a daunting assignment from God: she would
be the mother of the Savior with no human father, so she
would be disgraced in the eyes of her neighbors, who would see only
a pregnant teenager with no husband. Her response was complete
surrender. She saw herself as the Lord's servant. Her identity came
completely from him, so she wasn't oppressed by fear of what people
would think.

Responding to God's assignments with complete surrender is
a high calling, and yet that is what God asks of us. Sometimes we
don't have complete information, but only the next step. Sometimes
the assignment isn't something we would choose. Sometimes, as in
Mary's case, the Lord takes us completely out of our comfort zones.
In all these circumstances, faith asks for the surrender of our agenda
and the embrace of God's.

In what area do you need to surrender to God today? There is
vast freedom in surrendering to the Lord. Trusting him leads to the
peace that enabled Mary to follow through on all God asked of her. He
promises the same peace to us.

FOOD FOR THOUGHT

Surrender to God's agenda, and freedom will follow.

THE WHOLE POINT

Let love be your highest goal!

—*1 Corinthians 14:1 NLT*

It's important to have goals for your life. But if you set your goals without love, then people become projects. You will use them to get to your goals. And you will miss the whole point of life, because the whole point is learning how to love.

So bring love into the equation. Don't say, "I want my family to stop the unhealthy practices that have become such a negative influence." That's a goal that requires you to fix your family. Instead say, "I want to provide daily healthy meals for my family. I want to be a more cheerful, grateful person to live with. I want to support my family in their health goals this year." If your family isn't completely on board with The Daniel Plan in the beginning, treating them with love rather than as projects will be the most helpful course of action.

What loving goal could you set for yourself? God is eager to empower you to fulfill it.

FOOD FOR THOUGHT

Incorporating love into your goals will make you a powerful force for good in your relationships.

PRAYING FOR US

In the same way, the Spirit helps us in our weakness. We do not know what we ought to pray for, but the Spirit himself intercedes for us through wordless groans. —Romans 8:26

The Holy Spirit helps us with our daily problems. He even helps us pray. We can say, "Lord, this is so big I don't even know how to pray for it. All I have is this inner groaning, this longing to change. I don't know what I need, but you do. Holy Spirit, please pray for me. I so much want to become the person you made me to be."

Don't be afraid to let the inner groaning come up. Let the Spirit pray for you while you are quiet. You may get words to ask for something. Maybe you'll just say, "Lord, I trust you. Help me." Or you may get no words. No problem. The Spirit knows what you need. How amazing it is that the Holy Spirit is praying for you right now.

FOOD FOR THOUGHT

Be still and be confident that he always helps you in your weakness.

NEW BEGINNINGS

The LORD had said to Abram, "Go from your country, your people and your father's household to the land I will show you."

—*Genesis 12:1*

God told Abram (Abraham) to leave the place and the people he was familiar with and go to completely unfamiliar territory. It took tremendous faith and courage for him to say yes to such dramatic changes in his life. But the blessings God had in store for Abram and his descendants would happen only if he was willing to endure change.

Likewise, making changes on The Daniel Plan—changing the way you eat, the way you exercise, or the way you think—can feel as disruptive as going to a new country. It can feel like leaving behind the family in which you grew up. Yet the blessings God has in store for you and those close to you will happen only if you choose the faith and courage to say yes to change.

FOOD FOR THOUGHT

There are rich rewards when you have the courage to say yes to new beginnings and take steps of faith like Abraham.

QUICK TO LISTEN

Everyone should be quick to listen.

—*James 1:19*

How can we show love and honor and support to each other through the challenge of getting healthy? One way is to listen to each other. James urges us to seek first to understand (by listening) and only then try to be understood. Listening includes paying attention to the other person's body language and tuning in to their emotions.

A proverb goes even further, urging us to listen carefully to wise people who speak correction into our lives: "Like an earring of gold . . . is the rebuke of a wise judge to a listening ear" (Proverbs 25:12).

Who do you know who needs a good listening ear? Is there someone in your small group, family, or circle of friends who can't seem to get a word in edgewise? Who can you show love by asking, "How are you really doing?" and then listening to their answer? Become a safe person who is willing to listen without judgment to the challenges others struggle with. One of the greatest gifts you can offer someone is your listening ear.

FOOD FOR THOUGHT

By learning to listen with your heart, you can become a tremendous blessing to the people around you.

GOD'S ABUNDANT FEAST

Then God said, "I give you every seed-bearing plant on the face of the whole earth and every tree that has fruit with seed in it. They will be yours for food."
—Genesis 1:29

When God made Adam and Eve, he gave them an abundant array of plants to nourish their bodies. Plant foods are full of nutrients our bodies need for health. Dr. Mark Hyman says that the power of plants runs important functions in your body—food truly is medicine.

If you're not used to eating fruits and vegetables, you'll be amazed that your tastes will actually change the more you choose real foods. As you increasingly eat real food, your cravings for sugar and manufactured foods will be replaced by deep satisfaction from naturally sweet things. Experiment with a fruit or vegetable you've never tried before. Treat it as a taste of the Garden of Eden.

FOOD FOR THOUGHT

Every fruit and vegetable on the planet is nourishing, life-giving food for you to enjoy. It has the power to transform your health.

LEVEL WITH EACH OTHER

We will speak the truth in love, growing in every way more and more like Christ.
                                                    —*Ephesians 4:15 NLT*

If we want to support each other in health, we need to be able to level with each other. We have to love somebody enough to speak the truth, and we have to love somebody enough to *receive* the truth from him or her. The Bible says, "Better is open rebuke than hidden love. Wounds from a friend can be trusted" (Proverbs 27:5–6). When somebody truly loves you, they won't be afraid to tell you what you need to hear, not just what you want to hear.

When you speak the truth, do it in love—not in anger, pride, self-righteousness, or judgment. It's so much easier for someone to hear the truth when it is conveyed with humility, kindness, and genuine concern. This kind of honesty will lead you into true, Christ-centered community.

Biblical fellowship involves deep commitment out of genuine love for one another. Leveling with each other will help our spiritual and emotional growth, and even our physical transformation.

FOOD FOR THOUGHT

The deeper the conversation, the deeper the friendship. Truth conveyed with love is a powerful gift.

POWER OF FORGIVENESS

Be kind and compassionate to one another, forgiving each other, just as in Christ God forgave you. —Ephesians 4:32

If we want to show real love and support to each other, we will free each other from the burden of blame by offering forgiveness. We'll cut each other slack, letting go of the other person's failures and treating others as Jesus treats us. Jesus prayed even for those who were killing him: "Father, forgive them, for they do not know what they are doing" (Luke 23:34).

Our job is not to make people feel badly for their mistakes. Our job is to reach out to them when they fall and help them get back up on their feet. Our job is to say, "Hey, I know you're having a tough time, but I believe in you. I know you can do this. I'm here to help you." Nothing is more liberating than to know that somebody believes in you.

Who in your small group, family, or workplace needs you to offer them the grace of forgiveness and understanding?

FOOD FOR THOUGHT

Offer someone grace and forgiveness, and you will nourish their heart and soul while rejuvenating your relationships.

MAKING IT FOR THE LONG HAUL

I discipline my body like an athlete, training it to do what it should.
—*1 Corinthians 9:27 NLT*

Does it surprise you that the apostle Paul trained his body and not just his soul? Paul needed to be in shape, because his ministry required great physical stamina. He logged thousands of miles of travel on foot, taking the gospel from town to town. Paul didn't have horses or wagons to ride, so he literally walked across what is now Turkey, up and down mountains and a high plateau.

Paul compared his life to a race he was running, and he ran each step with purpose. We, too, need the stamina to run the race God has planned for us. You can't do anything on this earth without your body; good health keeps it running efficiently. That means we need to practice healthy habits that build strength.

How could you incorporate more movement and strength training into your life? Or is there another area in The Daniel Plan you'd like to focus on this week that will build your physical, emotional, or spiritual endurance?

FOOD FOR THOUGHT

Caring for your body's health will help you remain strong in all the areas where God has called you.

NOTHING CAN SEPARATE US

I am absolutely sure that not even death or life can separate us from God's love.
　　　　　　　　　　　　　　　　　　　　　—*Romans 8:38 NIrV*

Not even the worst times of our lives can separate us from God's love. Certainly our mistakes can't separate us. The habits we learned as children can't separate us. Our failed attempts to get healthy can't separate us. Our fears for today, our worries for tomorrow, or wherever we are emotionally—nothing will be able to separate us from the love of God demonstrated by our Lord Jesus when he died for us.

Isn't that a wonderful promise? It is the foundation on which we base everything we do, every change we make, every new habit we develop—that God's love will never stop. There are many uncertainties in your future, but there is one thing that is certain, and that is God's love for you.

What are the things you have feared might separate you from God's love? Write down each one. Then write down this truth about them: "This can't come between God and me. Jesus will redeem even this."

FOOD FOR THOUGHT

Nothing can come between God's love and you.

GOD GIVES REST

It is useless for you to work from early morning until late at night, just to get food to eat. God provides for those he loves even while they sleep.
—Psalm 127:2 NIrV

Working from early morning until late at night is not God's deepest desire for you. So if you have long work hours, ask him to intervene so that you can get enough rest. Maybe the most spiritual thing you can do today is take a nap!

Sometimes we don't rest well because we are anxious about our circumstances. If anxiety hinders you from rest, deliberately cast your cares onto God. Tell him what is troubling you. If you have difficulty letting go, try this: hold your hands out, palms down, and picture yourself putting your concerns into God's hands. Psalm 4:8 expresses this confidence that you could commit to memory: "In peace I will lie down and sleep, for you alone, LORD, make me dwell in safety."

What will it take for you to get enough rest this week? Consider making your sleep routine a priority and taking short breaks for replenishment during the day.

FOOD FOR THOUGHT

Adequate rest will equip your body and mind with the strength to fulfill all that God calls you to.

PROTECTING YOUR BODY

No one ever hated their own body, but they feed and care for their body, just as Christ does the church.   —*Ephesians 5:29*

There are four ways you can treat your body. First, you can *reject* it, which a lot of people do. "I don't like my body. Give me another model." They treat it like it's a mistake. Second, you can *neglect* your body, which is what most of us do. We don't pay attention to what our bodies need. Third, you can go to the other extreme and try to *perfect* it. You can become narcissistic, wrapped up in how great you look. Your body becomes an idol.

The Bible says all three of these attitudes are off target. Instead, the Bible invites you to *protect* your body. Protect your health. Why? Because God created your body, Jesus paid for your body, and the Holy Spirit lives in your body (1 Corinthians 6:19–20). God created you just the way he wanted you. He loves your body. It is God's gift to you. He invites you to join him in caring for what he has entrusted to you.

FOOD FOR THOUGHT

Protecting your body with food, exercise, and rest is a way of expressing gratitude to God for the gift of your body.

REBUILDING A DREAM

"If it pleases the king and if your servant has found favor in his sight, let him send me to the city in Judah where my ancestors are buried so that I can rebuild it." —Nehemiah 2:5

Nehemiah was a high-ranking official serving the king of Persia when God called him to go hundreds of miles to Jerusalem, a ruined city he had never seen, and rebuild it. When Nehemiah went, he faced obstacle after obstacle, including armed resistance from the people living near Jerusalem.

What is the dream God has laid on your heart? Even if it's as difficult as rebuilding a ruined city while defending against attackers, God can make it happen. You may have to deal with delay (Nehemiah did) and opposition and other challenges. But if it truly is from God, and you persevere, it will happen. "Commit your way to the LORD; trust in him, and he will do this" (Psalm 37:5).

Consider writing down the dream God has laid on your heart— and the first step you will take. This will take you one step closer to doing what it takes to bring your dream into reality.

FOOD FOR THOUGHT

Step out in faith, and enter the adventure of relying on God to fulfill your dream.

SHEDDING WHAT SLOWS US DOWN

Let us strip off every weight that slows us down, especially the sin that so easily trips us up. And let us run with endurance the race God has set before us. —*Hebrews 12:1 NLT*

The writer of Hebrews compares the life of faith to a race. He wants us able to run that race with endurance, not quitting the moment it gets tiring. Endurance builds over time, with daily practice. Endurance is also much easier if we strip off any weights that slow us down, such as distractions and habits of sin. Whatever holds us back from running the race God has set before us needs to be put aside.

Think of the goals you have set for yourself. What distractions are getting in the way of those goals? What habits are less than beneficial? You might concentrate on just one distraction at a time. Resolve by God's grace to leave it behind. Simplify your life and only do what really counts.

FOOD FOR THOUGHT

When we strip off the weights that slow us down, we can run God's race with so much more vitality.

WHY WE DO WHAT WE DO

So whether you eat or drink or whatever you do, do it all for the glory of God.
—*1 Corinthians 10:31*

It takes energy to forge new habits. Energy comes from motivation. The "why" determines how long you will persevere in pursuing a prize. The reason determines your motivation.

Here are two truths to remember when you feel like giving up. First, remember the reason you're getting healthy—you're doing it for the glory of God. He cares about your health because he wants to use your life to change the world.

Second, remember the reward: better physical health, more strength and energy, a sharper mind, deeper friendships, and stronger faith. Focus on your purpose, not your problems. Obstacles are what you see when you take your eyes off the goal. If you want to accomplish your goals, remember the reason and the reward.

What is a new habit you want to adopt? What is your reason? Your reward?

FOOD FOR THOUGHT

Aiming for glorifying God will give you the strength to persevere in your journey toward health.

FRIDAY

PUT THE PAST
BEHIND YOU

One thing I do: Forgetting what is behind and straining toward what is ahead, I press on toward the goal to win the prize for which God has called me heavenward in Christ Jesus. —*Philippians 3:13–14*

One of the main hindrances that keeps people from becoming what God wants them to become is their past. People often struggle to overcome past hurts and patterns of behavior.

Don't let your past distract you. Your past is past. Today is a brand-new day. Maybe you've had some setbacks. Maybe you've been knocked down dozens of times. That's normal. You can still get back up and keep going. That's what winners do: they get back up and run for the finish line, no matter how many times they stumble. They're focused.

Consider talking out your memories with a friend who will listen and not judge. Ask them to pray for you. Then, if you feel stuck on something in your past, think about how God sees you now: he forgives your past, calls you his beloved, and promises to complete the good work he has begun in you. Don't let your past keep you from your future.

FOOD FOR THOUGHT

You are a new creation in Christ, and God has called you to a heavenly prize.

QUIET BREAKS

I was very worried. But your comfort brought me joy.

—Psalm 94:19 NIrV

At least once a day, go out in your backyard or close your office door or sit in your car, and be quiet for a few minutes, tuning into God. You could just silently sit in his presence, or you could meditate on a verse like Psalm 18:2, "The Lord is my rock, my fortress and my deliverer; my God is my rock, in whom I take refuge."

When you feel your pressure going up, stop and say, "God, I want to tune in to you again. I want to focus on you." Take these mini-breaks during the day to refocus on the greatness of God.

Maintaining new habits is hard, and stress can make you slip back into your old ways. You start thinking, *Maybe I should just coast for the next couple of months.* But coasting is a downhill journey! A five-minute break with God can recharge you and keep you moving onward and upward. When will you take a five-minute break today to be quiet before God?

FOOD FOR THOUGHT

A quiet break with God is a gift to recharge your body and your soul.

DEFEATING DOUBT

His compassions never fail. They are new every morning; great is your faithfulness. —*Lamentations 3:22–23*

How do you defeat doubt? When you begin to doubt yourself, remember three things:

First, remember God's goodness in the past. Make a list of all the things he's done in your life and just start being thankful. Write them down so you can see them. The very act of writing them imprints them on your mind.

Second, remember God's presence today. He's with you right now. You're not alone. He has promised, "Never will I leave you; never will I forsake you" (Hebrews 13:5).

And third, remember God's promises for tomorrow. There are thousands of them in the Bible. They're like blank checks that you can just write out: "God, I am claiming this one today." Knowing God's promises is a good reason to read your Bible daily.

God's goodness in the past, God's presence today, God's promises tomorrow. Doubt fades in this light. When discouragement arises or distractions get in the way, remind yourself of his faithfulness. His mercies begin afresh each morning.

FOOD FOR THOUGHT

God promises, "I will strengthen you and help you; I will uphold you with my righteous right hand" (Isaiah 41:10).

COMMIT YOUR BODY TO GOD

Present your members as slaves of righteousness for holiness.
—Romans 6:19 NKJV

The apostle Paul urges the Romans to present their members (body parts) as slaves of righteousness. He wants them to offer each part of their bodies in devoted service to God. He wants them to commit everything to God—hands for making things, mouths for speaking, ears for listening, muscles for working—their whole bodies.

Committing your body to God is the starting point in getting your life on track. For change to happen in any area of your life—whether financial, vocational, educational, mental, or relational—it actually works best to begin with the physical. Why? Because your body affects your behavior. Your muscles affect your moods and your motivation. If your body feels weak, *you* feel weak.

Consider setting aside some time to present your body to God for his service. The Bible says you "are God's handiwork, created in Christ Jesus to do good works, which God prepared in advance for us to do" (Ephesians 2:10).

FOOD FOR THOUGHT

God wants to be Lord of your body. He bought it by the precious blood of Jesus and longs to use it for his glory.

LEAVE THE PAST BEHIND

"Forget the former things; do not dwell on the past."

—Isaiah 43:18

It's easy to say don't dwell on the past, but sometimes the past seems stubbornly present. You don't have to be stuck there. One thing you can do is tell your story to a trusted person who will listen and pray for you. Pray that the wounds of the past will heal rather than hold you back in the present. The Bible says, "Ask boldly, believingly, without a second thought" (James 1:6 MSG).

Another thing you can do is examine the ways the present is different from that painful past. Identify things that are different now, and thank God for them. Thank him for the good people in your life. Thank him for your church family or your small group. Thank him for the knowledge about how to be healthy that you have now. Thank him for the resources he's put in your life to help you change. Thank him for his love that never fails. He is with you now, delivering you from the prison of the past.

FOOD FOR THOUGHT

The past is past. Your future is in the hands of a loving God.

RESIST DISCOURAGEMENT

Let us not become weary in doing good, for at the proper time we will reap a harvest if we do not give up. —*Galatians 6:9*

How do you handle weariness? Why not rest—even nap—for a little while? Then get up to try again. Sometimes the best rest is in God's presence just soaking in his goodness. Being with people who love us can also recharge our batteries and ward off discouragement.

Discouragement is an enemy of our goals. To say, "It can't be done" is the opposite of saying, "I can do all this through him who gives me strength" (Philippians 4:13). We guard against discouragement by celebrating the small victories we have when we make good choices.

We all get discouraged at times. We may even become weary in doing good, especially if we hit a plateau where positive changes don't seem to be happening. At those moments, the apostle Paul offers encouragement: we truly will see blessing if we stick with it.

FOOD FOR THOUGHT

Regularly celebrating small victories and taking time to rest helps combat weariness and discouragement.

THANKFUL FOR FAITH

*Just as you received Christ Jesus as Lord, continue to live your lives in him,
rooted and built up in him, strengthened in the faith as you were taught,
and overflowing with thankfulness.* —Colossians 2:6–7

Faith is the foundation of The Daniel Plan, and God calls each of us to make it the foundation of our lives. The best thing about building our lives on a foundation of faith is that when life doesn't make sense, we can still have peace. There are moments on mountaintops and moments in deep valleys of despair. Even if everything on earth is broken, we can still have joy because of faith. Faith takes us beyond circumstances, beyond answers, and beyond what we see.

We can count on God to work actively in our lives, building our faith. Even the smallest bit of faith honors God, and he waters and nourishes it. What a beautiful gift! Thank God and let him strengthen your heart even more. Look for people, events in the world, and passages of Scripture that feed your faith.

FOOD FOR THOUGHT

The life of faith is what pastor and teacher Eugene Peterson called "a long obedience in the same direction,"[7] and it leads ultimately to a life overflowing with gratitude.

A NEW LIFE

If anyone is in Christ, the new creation has come: The old has gone, the new is here! —*2 Corinthians 5:17*

How great is a life in Christ! Our old life has passed away and a new life has begun. We're free of regrets, so we can move forward from the past into a new future that God has waiting for us. We need to reframe our thoughts around this idea of our new identity in Christ, that we are new people.

Do you experience yourself as a new person, or do old habits cling to you? Let the past go. Your new life has begun. In 1 Thessalonians 1:4, God says you are his chosen one, dearly loved. Do you live like a chosen and dearly loved person? Does that fill your mind so that it affects your emotions and choices? If not, meditate on 1 Thessalonians 1:4. Let it sink into your mind right now.

FOOD FOR THOUGHT

You are a new person. You belong to Christ; he chose you and dearly loves you.

LIGHT OF THE WORLD

You are the light of the world. A town built on a hill cannot be hidden.
—*Matthew 5:14*

God has chosen you to give light to the world by the way you live. This will happen more and more as you yield yourself to his transforming work inside you. Colossians 3:12 says you are chosen and dearly loved. John 15:15 says you are Christ's friend. Colossians 3:3 says you are hidden with Christ in God. These things are true about you right now based on God's work. They aren't based on anything you do or any goals you are trying to achieve.

If you wrap these verses around your heart and soul, you'll start to look at yourself differently and become able to pass this gift on to others. He surrendered his whole life on the cross—so that you could be forgiven, made new, made clean. There are no longer any barriers between you and God.

As you refocus your heart, mind, and life on this truth, you'll be able to move forward in all the ways that God has intended for you. He will make sure you shine as a light in a shadowed world.

FOOD FOR THOUGHT

You are a light, shining with the brightness of God.

THE THRONE OF GRACE

Let us then approach God's throne of grace with confidence, so that we may receive mercy and find grace to help us in our time of need.

—Hebrews 4:16

We can confidently draw near to God in the ups and downs of life. His throne is a place where we can receive mercy and find grace. As he promises in Hebrews, "Never will I leave you; never will I forsake you" (13:5). Nothing can separate us from his love.

Calling God's presence "the throne of grace" is so inviting. It lets us know we will receive a warm embrace from the King of Kings and the Lord of Lords. He accepts us wholeheartedly.

God has an everlasting love, backed by his mercy and grace. These are not things we need to earn. We find them as we approach his throne. There's nothing we need to do. There are no works to perform or hoops we need to jump through.

FOOD FOR THOUGHT

God's throne is a throne of grace. You can approach him with abundant confidence no matter what.

WITH ALL YOUR HEART

You will seek me and find me when you seek me with all your heart.
—Jeremiah 29:13

God promises us, once again, his presence. He's right there at any moment, offering us the gift of his loving presence before we even ask.

How do we seek him with all of our hearts? Establishing a few routines can make that happen. Our morning routine can involve some type of surrender and devotion before God. If you're not a morning person, you don't have to dedicate a full hour of prayer time. It's simply a time of bowing your heart before God, saying, "Lord, I devote this day to you, my heart, my life." This is a way to begin a surrendered day, following him wherever he leads.

Another way is to feed our souls with nourishment from the Bible. It is God's love letter to us, and he reveals himself through his Word. The psalmist says about God's Word, "The precepts of the LORD are right, giving joy to the heart" (Psalm 19:8).

FOOD FOR THOUGHT

It's a tremendous blessing to seek God with all our hearts. How replenishing it is when we make a practice of seeking him as part of our daily routine.

SHORT ACCOUNTS

*If we confess our sins, he is faithful and just and will forgive us our sins and
purify us from all unrighteousness.* —1 John 1:9

A good daily routine to consider is to keep an open channel of communication between you and God by confessing your shortcomings. This is called "keeping short accounts with God."

When we veer off course, if we bring our situation to God right away, we come back in alignment with him. He purifies us, miraculously removing all our impurities through his power. It's a freeing, gracious way to live.

We don't need to be perfect; we just need to be able to keep an open heart before him. We don't pretend to be something we're not, but instead bring who we are to God every day—the best and the worst of us, knowing that he will cleanse us.

God says, "Seek me and live" (Amos 5:4). We can seek him with our requests, our thanksgiving, and with our mistakes. We can seek him in all things, because he is faithful, just, and merciful.

FOOD FOR THOUGHT

Keep short accounts with God and you'll find that your communication with him is always open.

YOUR NEW IDENTITY

You did not choose me, but I chose you and appointed you so that you might go and bear fruit—fruit that will last. —John 15:16

How blessed you will be if you steep yourself in the Bible's truth about your new identity. Jesus has chosen you. You are wanted and included. He chose you to bear fruit, and he will make sure that the fruit grows by his grace.

Many other passages about your identity are good to meditate on. John 1:12 and Romans 8:14 say you are a child of God and God is your father. First Corinthians 6:17 says you are united to the Lord and are one with him in spirit. Ephesians 4:24 says you are righteous and holy. Take time with each of these truths, allowing them to settle deeply into your heart and influence the way you think.

You're not an orphan, because God has chosen you as his own child. You're not the sum of your mistakes, because God has declared you righteous and holy in his eyes. You're not hopeless, because God has redeemed your life through his Son. Let yourself believe these things.

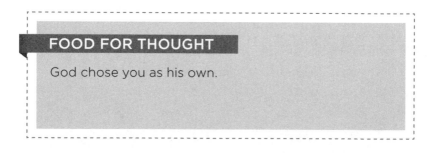

FOOD FOR THOUGHT

God chose you as his own.

CHOOSING STILL WATERS

The LORD is my shepherd. He gives me everything I need. He lets me lie down in fields of green grass. He leads me beside quiet waters. He gives me new strength. —Psalm 23:1–3 NIrV

What a visual picture this is of a loving shepherd who makes sure that we lack nothing, that we can feed on green pastures and drink still waters. Who doesn't want their soul to be restored?

To enter into this beautiful scene, we need to make a choice. The green pastures and still waters are always waiting for us. God's arms are always open wide, but we have to choose to enter into these peaceful moments. Those choices come in times of silence and solitude. We might take a five-minute break or have a great morning or evening prayer routine or carve out ten minutes before the kids get home from school or before an evening meeting. If we make this time to rest in God as our shepherd, he will certainly restore our souls.

FOOD FOR THOUGHT

In God's presence, he restores our souls and we lack no good thing.

RELYING ON HIS FAITHFULNESS

Teach me your way, LORD, that I may rely on your faithfulness.
—*Psalm 86:11*

It's hard sometimes to find rest for our souls. We may hit a season with tremendous challenges in it, and our hearts are naturally troubled. Yet God promises us a peace beyond our circumstances. In Psalm 145 the psalmist says, "The LORD is trustworthy in all he promises and faithful in all he does. The LORD upholds all who fall and lifts up all who are bowed down . . . The LORD is near to all who call on him . . . The Lord watches over all who love him" (vv. 13–14, 18, 20). He's faithful no matter what our circumstances are, no matter the depths of our struggles.

Who doesn't fall down? We all do. There's nothing to be ashamed about. Falling down is being human. The Lord will help us stand up again if we draw near to him. He promises that he's faithful.

FOOD FOR THOUGHT

In the tender seasons of our lives, God is always faithful to us.

FULLNESS OF JOY

You always show me the path of life. You will fill me with joy when I am with you. You will make me happy forever at your right hand.

—Psalm 16:11 NIrV

God has made known to us the path of genuine, abundant life. That means we don't need to figure it all out on our own, because he's paved the way in front of us. Every day we simply put one foot in front of the other. We are like the Israelites crossing the Red Sea, taking step after step in faith that the waters will stay parted and the ground will be dry.

Along this path, in his presence, there's fullness of joy. When the hard things come around, there's that choice to stay on the path, to put one foot in front of the other, to find joy in the midst of the chaos, to find his presence there with us.

At the end of the film *The Bucket List*, as one of the characters is passing away, he says, "I'm just going to ask you to do one more thing for me. Find the joy in your life." We can find the joy by taking those persistent steps of trust with God by our side.

FOOD FOR THOUGHT

God has fully given us joy in his presence; right next to him are pleasures forevermore.

REMAINING IN CHRIST

He cuts off every branch in me that bears no fruit, while every branch that does bear fruit he prunes so that it will be even more fruitful.

—*John 15:2*

God prunes us. He trims away parts of our lives that don't bear fruit. This is a great blessing: he moves obstacles and distractions so they don't get in the way of our growth. He also lifts and supports us in the areas that we need it.

Pruning may be painful, but it's essential for growth and health. "Remain in me, as I also remain in you. No branch can bear fruit by itself; it must remain in the vine. Neither can you bear fruit unless you remain in me" (John 15:4). Only by staying connected to God will we stay connected to true life. It's an active choice on our part to remain in him. Without him, we lose the source that sustains our growth. It's the only way to bear fruit.

FOOD FOR THOUGHT

Remaining in God, even when he prunes us, will lift and support us so we can bear much fruit and bring honor and glory to him.

RESILIENCE

We are hard pressed on every side, but not crushed; perplexed, but not in despair; persecuted, but not abandoned; struck down, but not destroyed.
—2 Corinthians 4:8–9

Resilience means that no matter what our circumstances are, we are able and eager to try again. If we haven't eaten well for breakfast, we start over at lunch. If we've made a choice we regret, we begin with a new choice the next day. To be resilient like this, we need to cultivate acceptance and letting go: "It happened; now I move on."

No matter what happens at home, in the workplace, or in a relationship, we can use challenges as opportunities to strengthen our resolve and increase our awareness.

Setbacks are inevitable, disappointments and failures happen, but what defines us is how we respond. Henry Ford said, "Failure is simply the opportunity to begin again, this time more intelligently."[8]

Resilience relies on the bigger picture—God is the one in control. And if we trust him, no effort is wasted or useless. He supports us as we follow him. That's all the motivation we need to get back up and keep going.

FOOD FOR THOUGHT

When a setback happens, a resilient heart asks God for a fresh take, a fresh measure of grace, of love, and of power to keep going.

REMEMBERING HIS DEEDS

I will remember the deeds of the LORD; yes, I will remember your miracles of long ago. —Psalm 77:11

When we're trying to reframe our thoughts in more positive ways, one of the best things we can do is think about the deeds of the Lord. First of all, we think of the good and faithful things he has done in history, the things the Bible tells us about: making human beings, laying out a plan to redeem humanity, calling Israel to be his chosen nation, freeing the people from slavery in Egypt, sending his Son to become a man to live and die for us, raising Jesus from the dead—all of those great deeds in Scripture can remind us what a great God he has always been.

Second, we can remember what he's done in our lives. He called us out of sin into a relationship with him. He has provided for us in numerous ways.

In Joshua 4:1–7, Joshua tells the Israelites to make a monument of twelve stones to remind them of how God parted the Jordan River so they could cross on dry ground. We need remembrance stones like these in our own lives. What deeds of the Lord do you remember?

FOOD FOR THOUGHT

Remembering God's goodness and focusing on what he has done changes our thoughts and our attitude.

COME A LITTLE CLOSER

Come near to God and he will come near to you.

—*James 4:8*

What a beautiful invitation to get close to God. He is a great and holy God, yet he doesn't stand far off from us. He welcomes us just as we are, even with our limitations. All we need to do is take a step toward God, and he's already right there.

Any true relationship involves getting close enough to someone to be vulnerable with them. We need to get close enough to God that our weaknesses are laid bare and, in that, discover the glorious experience of his love touching those tender places.

We have the full assurance of his open arms whenever we approach him. We can confide in him exactly what is on our minds. Even if no one else understands the things we can hardly put into words, God understands and is glad to receive what we offer him.

Our responsibility is to take that step toward him. Then he steps toward us and immerses us in his goodness, his love, his mercy, and his grace.

FOOD FOR THOUGHT

God is always available and ready to meet with you.

THE GREATNESS

I also pray that you will understand the incredible greatness of God's power for us who believe him. This is the same mighty power that raised Christ from the dead and seated him in the place of honor at God's right hand in the heavenly realms. —Ephesians 1:19–20 NLT

How would our lives change if we really knew God's vast power? This incredible power raised Jesus from the dead! And it's available to us. His power has parted rivers so that people walked through on dry ground. His power turned water into wine—in fact, it's his power at work every time grape vines turn rain into grape juice. His power keeps the earth rotating around the sun at just the right speed and just the right angle. His power is at work all around us if only we would pay attention.

If we really believed in his power, we would be bold in offering his love and truth to other people. If we really trusted his power, we would pursue the goals he's given us with the confidence that he will turn dreams into reality.

With God, today's impossibility is tomorrow's miracle. Are you ready for one? Put your trust in his power, not your own willpower.

FOOD FOR THOUGHT

God loves you so much that he freely gives you his power to work in your life.

FRIDAY

MIGHTY WARRIORS

*Then the Israelites retreated, but Eleazar stood his ground and struck
down the Philistines till his hand grew tired and froze to the sword.*
—2 Samuel 23:9–10

King David spent decades fighting Israel's enemies, and the
cream of his army were the men known as his mighty warriors
(2 Samuel 23:8). These men took on the most impossible missions.
Eleazar, for instance, stood his ground when the rest of the Israelites
retreated from the battlefield. Picture him fighting alone, stroke after
stroke, until his hand muscles stiffened and froze to his sword.

That's a picture of what it's like to be Daniel Strong: pursuing
excellence in body and spirit, persevering against the odds, having the
physical and mental strength to fight on, even when others quit. We
don't get that way simply by trying harder; we need God's Holy Spirit
to fill us to accomplish such feats. The Bible says, "It is God who arms
me with strength and keeps my way secure" (Psalm 18:32).

FOOD FOR THOUGHT

God wants to bless you with the perseverance of
Eleazar and the strength of David's mighty warriors.

INTENTIONAL LIVING

My choice is you, GOD, first and only. And now I find I'm your choice!
—*Psalm 16:5 MSG*

God invites us to intentional living. So many circumstances are out of our control each day, but so many other things are within our control. For instance, we control aspects of our schedules, those little bits of free time here and there. We can be intentional about planning times of restoration and rest. We can be intentional about the times we draw near to God, bringing all of our hearts and souls to him.

God has chosen us, and he warmly invites us to choose him. Have you? In Psalm 16:8 (NIrV), the psalmist says, "I keep my eyes always on the LORD. He is at my right hand. So I will always be secure." That's what intentional living does: it keeps our eyes on the Lord so that we're not shaken by the difficult circumstances that inevitably come our way.

How will you choose God today?

FOOD FOR THOUGHT

God has chosen you, and he yearns for you to choose him.

INTO GOD'S PRESENCE

Since we have a great High Priest who rules over God's house, let us go right into the presence of God with sincere hearts fully trusting him. For our guilty consciences have been sprinkled with Christ's blood to make us clean, and our bodies have been washed with pure water.

—Hebrews 10:21–22 NLT

We never have to hang back from entering God's presence because we feel we aren't good enough. We never have to be embarrassed to approach him. We can go to him with awe and humility because he's a majestic King. And we can go to him with boldness because he has called us his own.

God invites us to come near to him with sincere hearts and sure faith because we have been cleansed from all of our sins. He sees us as new, fresh. We can come forth and exchange our earthly identity for his eternal one.

What do you want to say to God today? You don't have to censor your thoughts and feelings. He longs to hear whatever is on your heart.

FOOD FOR THOUGHT

Jesus is our High Priest who has made us worthy of welcome in his Father's presence.

PONDERING VS. WORRYING

Simeon blessed them and said to Mary, his mother: "This child is destined to cause the falling and rising of many in Israel, and to be a sign that will be spoken against, so that the thoughts of many hearts will be revealed. And a sword will pierce your own soul too."　　　　　—Luke 2:34–35

Mary had a new baby, and a wise old man named Simeon gave her a prophecy about the boy. It wasn't a comforting prediction: Jesus would be "spoken against," and a sword would pierce Mary's soul. Simeon didn't tell her that Jesus would die young and in agony while she watched, but he told her enough to upset her if she was inclined to worry.

The Bible tells us, though, that instead of worrying about the things that happened when Jesus was a baby and a growing child, Mary treasured them up and pondered them in her heart (Luke 2:19, 51). She reflected on them in light of her knowledge of God's goodness. Her complete surrender to God made her the perfect mother for the Savior.

What source of worry can you begin to offer to God?

FOOD FOR THOUGHT

Treasuring what we know about God's goodness is a key to peace.

SECURE HOPE

Let us hold firmly to the hope we claim to have. The God who promised is faithful. —Hebrews 10:23 NIrV

Isn't that great news? Our hope can be a confident expectation of getting what God has promised us. Hope in him will not disappoint us (Romans 5:5) because that kind of hope is in someone bigger than ourselves, bigger than whatever circumstances we're in the middle of here and now. God will do what he promised: transform us into the likeness of his Son (Romans 8:29).

All of God's promises are faithful and true. They are like life preservers that keep us afloat no matter what. Nothing can deflate them. Nothing can drown them. God's promises are far more stable than our circumstances or our feelings. His character is pure love, and we can count on that. No matter what's going on in our lives, we can cling to the hope that we profess and weather any storms that life brings. He promises, "I will uphold you with my righteous right hand" (Isaiah 41:10).

FOOD FOR THOUGHT

Place your hope on the solid rock of God's trustworthy promises.

SURPASSING KNOWLEDGE

I pray that you, being rooted and established in love, may have power, together with all the Lord's holy people, to grasp how wide and long and high and deep is the love of Christ, and to know this love that surpasses knowledge. —Ephesians 3:17–19

We all know how powerful love is. Human love can give us the courage to try something new. Human love can melt our hearts. Human love is what helps a baby grow into a loving, confident adult. Just imagine, then, how much more motivating, inspiring, and fulfilling God's love is.

Christ's love is greater than anyone can ever know. Here's how vast it is: there will never be a moment in your life when God is not loving you. You cannot make him stop loving you, because his love is based on his character. Isn't that so freeing? It doesn't depend on you. It's not about how well you're doing with your goals, at work, or in your relationships. It's not about how well you're doing, period.

Bask in his love, and let it move you. Resolutions are never enough to change the human heart. Heart transformation requires the love of God inside you, actively changing you.

FOOD FOR THOUGHT

God's love is the foundation for heart transformation.

ALL THINGS ARE POSSIBLE

"With man this is impossible, but with God all things are possible."
—Matthew 19:26

Pastor Rick Warren says, "It's hard to be spiritually strong and mentally alert when we're emotionally stressed or physically fatigued." That's why we want our bodies to be fit—not as an end in itself, but so we can possess the vitality to embrace all that God has for us.

God wants to work through us, spreading the peace of his kingdom and offering love to our neighbors. We need to be able to think creatively and pour ourselves out in relationships. Those activities take energy. Eating well and incorporating more movement into our day replenishes our reserves, enabling us to do what would have been impossible in a depleted state.

Sometimes we depend on God for so many things in our spiritual lives, our marriages, our finances, our ministries, but we haven't yet let him be involved with our physical health. The Daniel Plan is here to help us understand that getting healthy starts with drawing near to God, building our health on a foundation of faith.

FOOD FOR THOUGHT

When your trust is truly in God, nothing is out of your reach.

ABOVE AND BEYOND

Now to him who is able to do immeasurably more than all we ask or imagine, according to his power that is at work within us, to him be glory in the church and in Christ Jesus. —*Ephesians 3:20–21*

This is the theme verse of The Daniel Plan. It's all about God's power working in our lives.

The key to a faith-filled life is not trying harder or psyching ourselves up, but relaxing in God's grace. It's being filled with his power so that he can do through us all that he has designed us to do.

We have so many dreams, yet life can get in the way. Thankfully, we can look to God for his strength. As Paul says in Philippians 4:13, we can do all things through him who gives us strength. Or in Matthew 19:26, Jesus says, "With man this is impossible, but with God all things are possible." So many things that seem out of reach are possible with God.

What do you need God's power for? To improve your health, learn a new way to eat, move in different ways, improve your mental focus, deepen your faith? It's all possible through him.

FOOD FOR THOUGHT

God is able to do immeasurably more than you can imagine. To him be glory!

SATURDAY

THE HEART OF
THE WISE

The heart of the wise is in the house of mourning.

—*Ecclesiastes 7:4*

When bad things like loss and failure happen, we need to look squarely at them and acknowledge how they affect us. If the loss is big enough, we need a friend for support and validation, saying, "Tell me more about it." "That must have been so hard." "How does that feel?" When we feel their love for us, we find more strength to face what really happened.

The bigger the loss, the more we need people around us. Job suffered a series of terrible losses—his children died, he lost his health, he lost his livelihood—and the Bible says his three friends sat with him for seven days in silence (Job 2:11–13). That's a gift of comfort. Sometimes friends don't need to say anything; they just need to be present.

FOOD FOR THOUGHT

The most valued friends are often "those who, instead of giving advice, solutions, or cures, have chosen rather to share our pain and touch our wounds with a warm and tender hand" (Henri Nouwen).[11]

THE POWER OF THE SUN

He has identified us as his own by placing the Holy Spirit in our hearts as the first installment that guarantees everything he has promised us.
—2 Corinthians 1:22 NLT

God made the sun. It produces more power in one second than the human race has used throughout all of history. It has enough energy to burn for five billion more years.[12] And it's just one of the stars God made. That's how much power he has at his disposal.

God is the one who gives us the ability to move forward. He has commissioned us and identified us as his own. The Spirit, not our own power, is what equips us for God's service. This is the key to not giving up when we get tired. The Bible says, "It is God who works in you to will and to act in order to fulfill his good purpose" (Philippians 2:13).

When God gives you the will and the power to do something, you'll be able to do it. He will never ask you to do something without giving you the power to accomplish it. And his power is unlimited. He says, "I will empower you if you trust me."

FOOD FOR THOUGHT

God says, "Look to me. Draw near to me. My power is limitless, and I desire to freely give it to you."

THE LORD DETERMINES OUR STEPS

We can make our plans, but the LORD determines our steps.
—Proverbs 16:9 NLT

God doesn't just offer advice from the sidelines. When we commit ourselves fully to him, the Holy Spirit comes into our lives to direct and empower us. He wants us to let him determine our steps.

As we make changes in health habits that glorify him—changes about food or fitness or any other area—God has a part, and we have a part. Pastor Rick Warren likes to say, "You work it out, and God works it in." He provides the strength and guidance, and we rely on him rather than ourselves. At the same time, we still have to make a choice every moment to move forward on the path he has laid out. We have to choose to use the strength he offers. Day in and day out, we choose to make the small decisions that add up to big results. He will guide each step and keep us on his path.

FOOD FOR THOUGHT

God hasn't just laid out a good path for you to follow; he guides you on it.

MADE REALLY WELL

For you created my inmost being; you knit me together in my mother's womb. I praise you because I am fearfully and wonderfully made.
—Psalm 139:13–14

You don't need to look different in the mirror, have a different waist measurement or a different number on the scale. You are, right now, fearfully and wonderfully made. You are of great value to God.

"Even to your old age and gray hairs I am he, I am he who will sustain you. I have made you and I will carry you; I will sustain you and I will rescue you" (Isaiah 46:4). Neither gray hair nor anything else matters, because God chooses you, loves you, and sustains you.

Consider standing in front of a mirror and praying to have eyes to see yourself as he sees you. Pray to know that you are fearfully and wonderfully made. Ask him for the faith to believe that he treasures you just as you are.

FOOD FOR THOUGHT

God knit you together to be the person you are right now, a miracle in his sight.

THE IMPORTANCE OF STUMBLING

For you have delivered me from death and my feet from stumbling, that I may walk before God in the light of life. —Psalm 56:13

Pastor Rick Warren says, "When things have been hard and challenging, God promises to turn our stumbling blocks into stepping stones, crucifixions into resurrections." The very thing that seems difficult—a new way of eating, the challenge of exerting yourself in daily movement, a stressful relationship, a difficulty at work—can give God access to your heart and teach you more about yielding to him in everything.

When we step into potholes that we didn't anticipate, when some terrain brings significant loss and great grief, that's when we rush to God and say, "Deliver me, so that I can walk before you in the light of life. Turn this crucifixion experience into an opportunity for resurrection." God will respond; our job is to cultivate hope and keep moving ahead in his strength.

What at first seems like nothing but a stumbling block can be what helps us become more alive and more like Christ.

FOOD FOR THOUGHT

God wants to turn your toughest challenge into a cause for gratitude when he delivers you.

UNLIKELY REJOICING

We also glory in our sufferings, because we know that suffering produces perseverance; perseverance, character; and character, hope. And hope does not put us to shame, because God's love has been poured out into our hearts through the Holy Spirit, who has been given to us.

—Romans 5:3–5

Rejoicing in the face of problems doesn't come naturally to us. Yet the apostle Paul promises three big gifts that trials bring to us: perseverance, character, and hope.

Perseverance is the ability to do something hard for a long time. Some people are easy to love, but others take more effort. Emotional endurance gives us the fortitude to keep offering love to a neighbor even when it's not easy. So if we respond well to a trial, it can actually build in us the emotional muscle to love others more consistently. Paul calls that ability to love consistently "strength of character." It's being like Jesus. All of us who love God want to be more like his Son.

Finally, character strengthens our confident hope, our expectation that God will fulfill his promises. Hope is one of the biggest blessings God can give us.

Perseverance, character, hope—these are three surprising benefits of persevering when we face trials.

FOOD FOR THOUGHT

Holocaust survivor Corrie ten Boom's sister said, "No pit is so deep that God is not deeper still."[13] He's hard at work to bless us with perseverance, character, and hope.

GRACIOUSNESS FOR HEALTH

Bear with each other and forgive one another if any of you has a grievance against someone. Forgive as the Lord forgave you.

—Colossians 3:13

We don't need perfect friends. Instead, healthy relationships happen between people who bear with each other, who are gracious about each other's faults. Healthy relationships are built by people who are quick to forgive one another as soon as a grievance arises. It may be necessary to muster the courage to tell the other person we are hurt and to talk through the situation so it's less likely to happen again. But even in confrontation, loving friends talk peacefully as we let go of any desire to make the other person pay. Instead of retaliating in anger, we go to the other person in humility and calm strength. And often there's no need even for that, because with minor offenses we can forgive without pointing out the other person's faults.

Jesus said, "Do not condemn, and you will not be condemned. Forgive, and you will be forgiven" (Luke 6:37). Is there someone you need to forgive?

FOOD FOR THOUGHT

Because we are grateful that the Lord has forgiven us, we are able to offer forgiveness freely to others.

A THOUSAND YEARS

Your beauty should not come from outward adornment, such as elaborate hairstyles and the wearing of gold jewelry or fine clothes.

—1 Peter 3:3

The temptation in our culture is to look at our bodies as ornaments. We ask, how do I get people to notice and appreciate me? But imagine that a thousand people decided to take The Daniel Plan seriously and address the core issues of discipleship and body care. Suppose, conservatively, that they each added a year of vitality to their lives by doing that. A year with the extra energy to serve the Lord wholeheartedly. That would add a thousand years of service to the kingdom of God simply because people viewed their bodies not as ornaments but as instruments for God to use. A thousand years to be good models for their children and grandchildren. A thousand years to reach out to those in need, to lead Bible studies, or to disciple others. Another thousand years of service if we all just take small steps to care for the bodies God has entrusted to us.

Let's devote our lives to serving our Father. Let's nourish our bodies so that we have the stamina to glorify him with them.

FOOD FOR THOUGHT

Your body is an instrument through which God wants to work in the world.

INVESTIGATE MY LIFE

Investigate my life, O God, find out everything about me.
—Psalm 139:23 MSG

Once we are in Christ, God doesn't look at our struggle as though he were a prosecuting judge. He looks at it as a physician looks for a cure for our sin sickness.

So instead of trying to measure up to what we think God demands of us, God is saying, "I'm going to help you overcome this thing that is hurting you." When we fail, being filled with the Spirit doesn't mean, "Lord, I promise I'll try harder." It means, "Lord, why did I fail? What was the motivation? What set me up?" Then we wait for God to reveal insight to us. "Well, see how you did this, or maybe you pushed this, or maybe it was shame." Whatever went wrong, now God is our partner in overcoming the obstacle or setback.

We fail physically, but it helps us mature spiritually, because God says, "Let me show you why you failed. And I still love you. You're still my son or daughter. I haven't left you alone. You're going to be okay."

FOOD FOR THOUGHT

Whenever we want to make a life change, the Holy Spirit will counsel us through it, comfort us when we fail, and empower us to succeed in the future.

GOD SEEKS US

The LORD looks out over the whole earth. He gives strength to those who commit their lives completely to him. —2 Chronicles 16:9 NIrV

We talk about seeking the face of God. Did you know that God seeks us, too? No matter what we are doing, he is looking on. He is looking for people who say, "This is my life. I'm going to dedicate it to him." Our lives may be very ordinary and unglamorous. They may be far from ideal in our eyes, but God is not inviting us to dedicate to him an ideal. He is asking us to dedicate our actual ordinary lives. He is able to accomplish astonishing things through them

He doesn't ask for perfection. He asks for commitment. He's looking for loyalty and dedication to doing his will in the world, loving our neighbors as ourselves. He's seeking servants and friends who will partner with him over the long haul, even when it's difficult. He doesn't ask us to be strong—he'll provide the strength if we provide the commitment.

FOOD FOR THOUGHT

God is searching us out, looking for hearts fully committed to him.

LAVISHED

See what great love the Father has lavished on us, that we should be called children of God!
                                                                    —*1 John 3:1*

The whole Trinity lavishes love on us. Our heavenly Father calls us his true children. Jesus Christ sacrificed his life for us. And in the Holy Spirit, love is within us.

We are people who are loved, loved, loved. The apostle Paul says, "And I pray that you, being rooted and established in love, may have power, together with all the Lord's holy people, to grasp how wide and long and high and deep is the love of Christ, and to know this love that surpasses knowledge—that you may be filled to the measure of all the fullness of God" (Ephesians 3:17–19). He wants us to know this love that surpasses knowledge, because only when we truly know it will we be able to struggle fruitfully toward change. We are surrounded by love, before us, above us, behind us.

FOOD FOR THOUGHT

God has lavished his love on us; we are his!

WHAT WE CONTROL

Under pressure, your faith-life is forced into the open and shows its true colors. So don't try to get out of anything prematurely. Let it do its work so you become mature and well-developed, not deficient in any way.

—James 1:3–4 MSG

Most of what happens around you is completely out of your control. But you do control two important factors: you control your response and you control how much you choose to trust God.

Viktor Frankl, a Jew, was sent to one of the Nazi death camps of World War II. Frankl later wrote that while he was a prisoner, the guards stripped him of everything he had. They took his identity, his family, his clothes, even his wedding ring. But no one could take from him his freedom to choose his response. He wrote, "They offer sufficient proof that everything can be taken from a man, but one thing: the last of human freedoms—to choose one's attitude in any given set of circumstances, to choose one's own way."[14]

What matters in life is not so much what happens to us, but what happens *in* us. We choose. God uses circumstances to change us, grow us, and make us more like Christ.

FOOD FOR THOUGHT

We become better when we choose to respond in faith and believe that every circumstance is a tool God will use to make us more like Christ.

QUENCHED!

But those who drink the water I give will never be thirsty again. It becomes a fresh, bubbling spring within them, giving them eternal life.

—John 4:14 NLT

We don't want to live this life thirsty. If we don't let God satisfy our thirst, then instead of loving people, we try to get them to satisfy our thirst. We can end up demanding things from them that they're not designed to fulfill. For instance, if we're living thirsty, instead of loving our kids and releasing them to be who God created them to be, we try to shape them into people who do what makes us proud. Or we choose a job that will make us feel like we matter.

When our thirst is met in God and we know he created us, loves us, enlisted us, and is empowering us, then we will seek first his kingdom and not our own. It is so much more fulfilling to be a part of accomplishing God's purposes than our own limited purposes that fall short of what God designed for us. Our limited purposes can never really satisfy our souls the way God can.

FOOD FOR THOUGHT

If we drink deeply of God's living water, then we'll be free to love others and do God's work in the world.

COMMITTED

How can I save Israel? My clan is the weakest in Manasseh, and I am the least in my family.
—Judges 6:15

In the book of Judges, God calls Gideon—a very ordinary young man—to lead Israel in defeating the Midianites, who are oppressing God's people. Gideon's flaws and weakness are clear for all to see. Cowardice is just one of his flaws at the beginning of the story. He also utterly doubts God's ability to use him. So it's plain that when he eventually wins battles, he does so by God's strength and not his own.

An anonymous person is said to have stated, "Biblical saints aren't good. They're committed." Gideon is a great example of this. He wasn't chosen for his goodness. God worked through him because once he found his courage, he saw God was with him. And he could commit to God's purpose, knowing he wasn't on his own.

God doesn't ask for perfection—in fact, he works well with weakness and mistakes. He only asks for commitment.

FOOD FOR THOUGHT

Commitment goes farther than any good intention.

STEP BY STEP

In all your ways submit to him, and he will make your paths straight.

—Proverbs 3:6

Growth happens through a steady stream of little choices. If you want to eat in a better way, if you want to take care of your body and exercise more, it takes a series of small choices that add up to big results. You make small choices at every meal or every time you lace up your sneakers.

The same thing is true with your soul. Spiritual health is built up day after day, experience after experience. That's why the Bible so often uses the metaphor of a path to follow step by step.

The beauty of adding food to your life that heals, nourishes, and satisfies you deeply is that bite by bite, it will shift your body and mind into a state where you naturally crave what makes you thrive and feel good. The same is true in the spiritual realm: small dedicated choices will gradually shift your soul to crave the presence of God, which makes you thrive.

FOOD FOR THOUGHT

Small choices add up to transformation, bite by bite and step by step.

MAGNIFICENT OBSESSION

Seek the Kingdom of God above all else, and live righteously, and he will give you everything you need. —Matthew 6:33 NLT

Seeking first the kingdom of God is the magnificent obsession that we are all called to pursue. It is the description of Jesus' whole life. He stated the thread that held his life together in John 6:38: "I have come down from heaven, not to do my will but the will of him who sent me." A life of surrender, doing the Father's will, is why he came. At the start of his ministry, when his disciples asked him how to pray, what did he pray? "Hallowed be your name, your kingdom come" (Luke 11:2). Near the end of his life, as he was praying in the Garden of Gethsemane, he still said, "Father . . . not as I will, but as you will" (Matthew 26:39).

The magnificent obsession with God's will can completely free you up when you realize you weren't created to make your parents proud of you. You weren't created to make your kids feel loved. You weren't created to make your spouse happy. You were created to do the will of God. The only audience that you're to please is God.

FOOD FOR THOUGHT

Seek God's will above everything else.

GOD'S ATTENTIVENESS

*The eyes of the LORD are on the righteous, and his ears are attentive to
their cry.* —Psalm 34:15

What expression do you think his eyes would have if you could see them? His eyes are like the eyes of the parent of a small child. His eyes are delighted in you and watchful for your well being. He is attentive to your cry like the mother of an infant. When you call to him for help, he hears you right away. He may not give you what you want, but he will always give you what you need. And he will always listen to you with his full attention, caring about what you have to say.

God pays attention to everything his children say, do, and need. You are never out of his sight. The Bible says, "The eyes of the LORD are on those who fear him, on those whose hope is in his unfailing love" (Psalm 33:18). Focus your hope on his unfailing love, because his eyes are always focused on you.

FOOD FOR THOUGHT

Put your hope fully in God, because his eyes and ears are fully attentive to all your needs.

LIVING SACRIFICE

I urge you, brothers and sisters, in view of God's mercy, to offer your bodies as a living sacrifice, holy and pleasing to God—this is your true and proper worship.
　　　　　　　　　　　　　　　　　　　　　　　　—Romans 12:1

Sometimes the big, one-time sacrifices are the easiest ones. We check them off, and they're out of the way. But God calls us to ongoing, living sacrifice. We offer what we eat for breakfast, lunch, and dinner to him. We offer our attention in prayer each morning and throughout the day. We offer our energy to serve him all day long. This is our true and proper worship, our moment-by-moment offering.

He is pleased with that living sacrifice no matter what the mirror or the scale says. He is delighted by us no matter what. We may think we have little to offer, but God sees a devoted heart as the most valuable sacrifice he could have.

How can you shape your day today as an all-day, moment-by-moment offering? What choices does he invite you to make? Will you be a living sacrifice?

FOOD FOR THOUGHT

An all-day, moment-by-moment offering of your body, mind, and heart is so pleasing to God.

FOR THIS TIME, THIS PLACE

If you remain silent at this time, relief and deliverance for the Jews will arise from another place, but you and your father's family will perish. And who knows but that you have come to your royal position for such a time as this?
—Esther 4:14

Esther was a Jewish girl forced into the king of Persia's harem. By God's sovereignty, the king chose her as his queen, but he remained a dangerous man to deal with. Esther's uncle told her about a plot to massacre the Jews; he wanted her to persuade the king to stop the plot. For Esther to go to the king without being summoned was to risk her life. Her uncle's argument was simple: God had made her queen for this very reason, to risk her life for her people.

We are rarely called to risk our lives in the service of God, but we all need courage to face our circumstances. Even making healthier choices takes courage, because we often need to overcome deeply rooted patterns of comfort. What courageous step is God asking you to take now?

FOOD FOR THOUGHT

God achieves glorious things through those with the courage to step into the unfamiliar.

INFINITELY MORE

Now to him who is able to do immeasurably more than all we ask or imagine … to him be glory in the church and in Christ Jesus throughout all generations, for ever and ever! —*Ephesians 3:20–21*

Change can feel daunting at times, depending on whatever challenges we face. Whether the change involves improving our health, addressing our weight, trying to eat or move in a different way, improving our mental focus, or deepening our faith, the key is to rely on God's power working in our lives. This is the secret to a faith-filled life. It's not in doing more. It's not in rising to the occasion every time. Instead, we say, "God, you've promised a power greater than mine, and I'm asking you to show up and show off in my life." Then we step back, watch what he will do, and let him have all the glory.

What do you dream that God would do through your life? If it seems impossible, that's okay. It should be impossible in your own strength. Let yourself dream, and let your dream motivate you to rely on his power more and more as you get healthy. You'll be amazed to see how far beyond your imagination God can go.

FOOD FOR THOUGHT

We cannot imagine all that God really can do through his mighty power in us.

THE GRATITUDE BOOST

Every time I think of you, I give thanks to my God.

—*Philippians 1:3 NLT*

Paul's thankfulness for his friends in Philippi is an excellent example for us to follow. Gratitude changes our mindset and helps us see what's good about others. What might happen in your relationships if you thanked God for your family members when you woke up every morning, if you thanked God for your co-workers when you walked in the front door, if you thanked him for your friends and your neighbors as you drove home? Don't think first of what you want to get from them; think of what God is giving you through them already. Even people you aren't naturally drawn to offer unexpected gifts.

Studies show that the more grateful you are, the happier you are.[15] Positive thoughts about people will actually release beneficial chemicals in your brain. And your relationships will go much better if you go into them with an attitude of gratitude.

FOOD FOR THOUGHT

Your happiness level will skyrocket if you take time to remember the good things about the people around you.

GREAT FAITHFULNESS

Yet this I call to mind and therefore I have hope: Because of the Lord's great love we are not consumed, for his compassions never fail. They are new every morning; great is your faithfulness. —Lamentations 3:21–23

Because of Israel's sin, God allowed the Babylonians to destroy Jerusalem and take its surviving population into captivity. The city was looted and burned. Its citizens died of war wounds and starvation. The temple was reduced to rubble. The prophet Jeremiah watched all this take place, and he wrote the poems in Lamentations to express his sorrow.

At the very center of the book, though, he wrote about his reason for hope despite the desolation. Although the suffering was terrible, he still dared to hope because he remembered the faithful love of God. God hadn't given up on his people. His faithfulness was too great; his mercy never failed.

No matter what you are going through, you can have hope for the same reason. God's faithful love never ends. His mercies never cease. He may allow loss and grief, but he will never abandon you. He longs for you to seek him as your greatest comforter.

FOOD FOR THOUGHT

You can dare to hope when you remember God's faithfulness. He will never forsake you.

CHOSEN

But you are a chosen people, a royal priesthood, a holy nation, God's
special possession, that you may declare the praises of him who called you
out of darkness into his wonderful light. —*1 Peter 2:9*

We all need to feel accepted. We need to belong. In fact, sometimes those longings can be mistaken for feeling hungry when we're really lonely or feeling unwanted. Maybe our parents were never satisfied with our grades or our appearance. Maybe our spouse or the people at work say critical things that cut us to the core. Those experiences make us doubt whether anybody anywhere truly accepts us as we are.

The great news is that God does accept us just as we are. You are a member of God's family. You belong. You're God's special possession. He didn't choose you because of how you look, what you do, or what family you were born into. He didn't choose you because of how many good things you do for your church or how successful you are as a parent. He chose you for you.

FOOD FOR THOUGHT

God chose you out of darkness, just as you are, to be part of his family.

COURAGEOUS CHANGE

Anyone who belongs to Christ has become a new person. The old life is gone; a new life has begun! —*2 Corinthians 5:17 NLT*

We all go through several stages when we change. Stage one is *not thinking* about changing. Not thinking about it at all. We can get locked into denial, rationalizing our behavior because we want to stay there. We can all relate to this at some point on our journey.

Stage two is thinking about changing. We read a book; we gather information. If you have gotten to stage two, you deserve applause for the effort it's taken to get to this stage. You're aware that your health could use improvement, and you're investigating how that might happen.

Stage three is planning. It is sitting down and creating an action step that is specific and measurable. Maybe we write down our goals to exercise for thirty minutes a day, three times a week. We mark our calendars with those appointments and begin to get into new routines with those life-giving habits.

Stage three isn't the end of the journey, but it's a solid beginning that deserves to be celebrated. We can't get to the stage of actually changing without these preliminary steps.

FOOD FOR THOUGHT

Real change takes time, and the early stages of thinking and planning are essential to the process.

ONE FOOT IN FRONT OF THE OTHER

*I'm staying on your trail; I'm putting one foot in front of the other. I'm not
giving up.* —*Psalm 17:5 MSG*

D r. Mark Hyman says that what you put on your fork dictates whether you are sick or well, slim or fat, depleted or energized. With all that riding on what you eat, it would be easy to feel overwhelmed. But there's no pressure to change instantly; gradual change over time is sustainable. Just put one foot in front of the other. There's plenty of grace while you are in the process. When you have a bad day, what matters is that you decide to get back on track and that you don't give up.

What do you tend to do when you have a bad day, when you feel lousy or you eat the wrong foods because you're busy or stressed? Be gracious with yourself, because God is gracious with you. Over time you will have more good days than bad ones, and the changes will be long-lasting for your health.

FOOD FOR THOUGHT

God is gentle with you while you are in the change process. The goal is progress, not perfection.

MAXIMIZING POTENTIAL

Let us therefore make every effort to do what leads to peace and to mutual edification.
—Romans 14:19

You will not make all the changes that you want by yourself. You need a group. That's why we encourage people to form small groups, comprised of friends who will be there with you through the ups and downs of life.

If you don't already have a group, who can you enlist? Is there someone at your workplace who might want to partner with you in getting healthy? Can you start or join a group at your church? Is there someone you can go walking with and pray with?

As members of God's family, we are designed to support each other. The words *mutual edification* in this verse mean to build each other up, to increase each other's potential. We can do that in many ways, such as by offering a listening ear when someone needs to talk, or by encouraging someone without judgment when they face a setback and feel like quitting. Let's remember to strengthen each other and help each other overcome the obstacles we face.

FOOD FOR THOUGHT

Imagine the improvements you can make if you find one or two people as your partners in better health.

NEW CLOTHES

Therefore, as God's chosen people, holy and dearly loved, clothe yourselves
with compassion, kindness, humility, gentleness and patience.
—*Colossians 3:12*

The reason we treat people with compassion, kindness, humility, gentleness, and patience is because of who we are: chosen, holy, and dearly loved. Healthy relationships grow out of a secure sense of our identity. If we are convinced that we are dearly loved, then that love spills over to other people. If we are conscious of having been chosen, then our ego takes a back seat to humility and putting others' interests ahead of our own. Our deepest needs for acceptance and significance have been met in God, so we can focus on compassion and kindness to others. And if we know we're holy, set apart for God's service, then patience toward others is the supernatural result.

Think of it: you are chosen, wanted, part of God's family. You are holy. You are dearly loved. Let it sink in. How will that affect your relationships today?

FOOD FOR THOUGHT

You can have healthy relationships because you are securely and permanently chosen, holy, and dearly loved.

DIVIDENDS

You need to persevere so that when you have done the will of God, you will receive what he has promised. —*Hebrews 10:36*

The final stage of the change process is maintenance—staying with the new behavior for at least six months. While it takes courage to begin to change, it takes endurance to stick with it. Scripture frequently praises the quality of endurance, because we need it so much. The apostle Paul says, "And let us not grow weary of doing good, for in due season we will reap, if we do not give up" (Galatians 6:9 ESV). If we practice endurance in the physical realm, it will train us for even more valuable endurance in the moral and spiritual realm. We will become more and more the kind of person that God designed us to be and others can count on.

God doesn't ask us to manufacture endurance on our own. He will give us the strength to endure if we ask for it. He also gives us friends to cheer us on.

FOOD FOR THOUGHT

Life is a marathon, and endurance pays big dividends. It makes your soul strong and enriches your relationships with God and others.

THE GOD OF HOPE

May the God of hope fill you with all joy and peace as you trust in him, so that you may overflow with hope by the power of the Holy Spirit.

—*Romans 15:13*

Even when our situation is full of challenges, we can confidently pray that the God of hope will fill us with the joy and peace that come from believing in him. He won't let us down. And in those moments when we feel we can't go any farther, placing our reliance wholly on him is crucial. We need the power of the Holy Spirit if we want to abound in hope. He is always right there, ready to help us when we ask.

God also asks for our participation in the process. We can integrate faith and fitness for maximum benefit because getting up and moving our bodies actually lifts our mood and alleviates anxiety, depression, and stress. Spending time with a friend is another way to connect with God's hope. Consider taking a brisk and prayerful walk with a friend. He often provides his arms of love through those closest to us.

FOOD FOR THOUGHT

Joy and peace come from the God of hope.

STAND UP AND WALK

Jesus said to him, "Get up, take up your bed, and walk."

—*John 5:8 ESV*

Jesus met a man who had been paralyzed for decades. The man lay on a mat near a pool of water. He told Jesus he wanted to be healed. Jesus did his part, and then the man had to fulfill his part of the healing: he had to obey Jesus by getting up, picking up his mat, and walking. Was it hard for the man to trust Jesus enough to stand on legs that hadn't worked for years? Even if it was, he overcame his fears and did something he'd never done before.

As important as it is to think about change and set goals, there comes a time when we have to move on to stage four of our change process: action. The time comes to trust Jesus and start walking a new way. We do something different—even small steps count. Go for it and take action, trusting Christ all the way.

FOOD FOR THOUGHT

If we heed Jesus' call to get up and walk, he promises to be with us every step of the way.

WRESTLING WITH GOD

Jacob replied, "I will not let you go unless you bless me."

—Genesis 32:26

Jacob had been through several hard decades of life when he faced an all-night wrestling match with an angel of God. Jacob needed to know that God was in his life and acting for his good, so he held on for all he was worth, refusing to let go until God blessed him.

We need that kind of determination in our faith. The Lord of the universe longs to see our tenacity. He doesn't want us to quit before the job is done. He is waiting for us to say, "No way, I'm not letting you go until you bless me, because I know you are a God of blessing and you are my true hope." If it's hard for you to hang on like that, then pray for the strength and patience to do it.

FOOD FOR THOUGHT

Hanging on to God pays off when we find our strength multiplied and our blessing overflowing.

FLESH MATTERS

The Word became flesh and made his dwelling among us.

—John 1:14

Jesus has a human body. There was a day in history when the infinite Son of God became a human being. He needed food and water and sleep. He went most places on foot, so he got tired. Eventually, he was brutally killed and rose from the dead with a body that was still human, though perfected. He still has that resurrected body now. He has gone back to be with the Father and the Holy Spirit in heaven and has taken his human body up into their shared divine life.

That's how much God values the body. He not only made your body, but he also took on a body much like yours for your sake. Whatever you're going through with your body, he knows what it's like. Your hands and feet, your core and your limbs—all of it—are precious to him beyond measure. Your body matters to God.

FOOD FOR THOUGHT

Out of love for you, the Son of God took on a human body for all eternity. That's how precious your body is to him.

THE BEST HARVEST

No discipline seems pleasant at the time, but painful. Later on, however, it produces a harvest of righteousness and peace for those who have been trained by it. —Hebrews 12:11

Exercise is a discipline. You have to do it regularly for it to be effective. Reading the Bible is a discipline. It, too, has to be done consistently if it is going to shape the way you think and act. Many people focus on the painful part of discipline, and they avoid it. But any kind of discipline, even physical discipline, produces a harvest of righteousness and peace.

Can physical discipline really help us become like Jesus? It can if we let it. If we prayerfully offer our food and exercise routines to him, he will use them to shape our souls as well as our bodies. We'll have more endurance and dependability in other areas of our lives. If we find joy in movement, that joy will spill over into the rest of our lives. We'll build our spiritual muscles along with our physical ones.

FOOD FOR THOUGHT

Discipline will reward you with righteousness and peace.

MORE THAN SPARROWS

Let your way of thinking be completely changed. Then you will be able to test what God wants for you. —*Romans 12:2 NIrV*

How do you talk to yourself? Do you say harsh things that you would never say to a friend? Some of us say cruel lies we've heard other people say to us, perhaps when we were children. The negative things people say often burrow deep and distort our thinking.

If you believe you're a "failure," you may think you're going to fail in your health goals. So success will be that much harder. It's important to replace false thoughts with true ones from God's Word. Jesus says you are enormously valuable to God: "Are not five sparrows sold for two pennies? Yet not one of them is forgotten by God. Indeed, the very hairs of your head are all numbered. Don't be afraid; you are worth more than many sparrows" (Luke 12:6–7). "See, I have engraved you on the palms of my hands" (Isaiah 49:16). When the discouraging thoughts come, replace them with the truth of God.

FOOD FOR THOUGHT

God has numbered the hairs of your head and engraved you on the palms of his hands.

THE POWER TO DO MORE

The power of the LORD came on Elijah and, tucking his cloak into his belt,
he ran ahead of Ahab all the way to Jezreel.　　　　*—1 Kings 18:46*

The prophet Elijah had a dangerous faceoff against the pagan priests of Baal. That day, God proved himself to be the only real God—he sent fire from heaven to light the offering on an altar. Having proved his point to the faithless King Ahab, Elijah ran the seventeen miles from Mount Carmel to Jezreel ahead of Ahab's horse-drawn chariot. Imagine outrunning a horse for seventeen miles!

Elijah didn't do it in his own strength, of course. So if you need strength to reach your fitness goals, pray for the power of the Lord to come on you. If, like Elijah, you are running to the glory of God, he will help you go the next leg of the race.

For what do you need the power of the Lord today? "Be strong and take heart, all you who hope in the LORD" (Psalm 31:24).

FOOD FOR THOUGHT

As you run for God's glory, may the power of the Lord come on you with every step so you can follow his will and finish the race strong.

SPIC AND SPAN

Do not call anything impure that God has made clean.

—*Acts 10:15*

The apostle Peter believed that Jesus had come as the Savior of the Jews. He and the other apostles assumed that if non-Jews wanted to get in on salvation, they had to convert to Judaism. To show Peter that Jesus was the Savior of non-Jews too, God sent Peter a vision. He showed him an array of animals that weren't kosher for Jews to eat, and he told Peter to eat them. When Peter expressed disgust, God said, "Do not call anything impure that God has made clean." In this way, Peter learned that anybody who believed in Jesus was made clean.

Today, we may not doubt our cleanness because of our ethnic background, but we may doubt it for other reasons. Some secret in our past. A number on the scale. A struggle with sin. But God says that if you believe in Jesus, you are made clean. He says it strongly. Don't call yourself impure. Your past is forgiven. Your present is covered in the blood of Jesus. Your future awaits you, with God opening his arms to you. You are clean.

FOOD FOR THOUGHT

Believe the truth about yourself: God has made you clean, fully forgiven, with a new identity in Christ.

BRAVE STEPS

Then Peter got down out of the boat, walked on the water and came toward Jesus. But when he saw the wind, he was afraid and, beginning to sink, cried out, "Lord, save me!" —Matthew 14:29–30

Peter overcame his fear enough to ask Jesus to tell him to walk on the water, too. When Jesus said, "Come," Peter actually had the courage to obey him and climb out of the boat. He walked for a while and then got distracted. That's when his fear took over again.

It's easy to blame Peter for becoming afraid, but think of how brave he was just to get out of the boat at all! His positive steps are worth celebrating. In the same way, it may be easy for you to blame yourself when you have gotten sidetracked from your goals and lost sight of Jesus. Instead of blaming yourself for those moments, focus on all the positive steps of faith you have made, and celebrate the small victories. Have you gotten out of the boat? Great! Have you gotten distracted and afraid? No problem—Jesus will help you get back on course.

FOOD FOR THOUGHT

When you walk on water, even for only a moment, celebrate that step of faith.

THE IT FACTOR

He who did not spare his own Son, but gave him up for us all—how will
he not also, along with him, graciously give us all things?

—*Romans 8:32*

If God loves you enough to send Jesus to die for you on the cross, why wouldn't he give you whatever else you need in life? Take a moment to think about God sending Jesus to die for you. Let it soak in that God did this for you. If he went to such an extreme measure for you, won't he give you the power to make good choices about your body as you continually look to him and draw upon his strength?

Yes, Philippians 2:13 says that God will give you both the power and the will to become all he intends for you to be. This is the factor not found in any secular fitness or health program. God's power, love, and grace is the "it" factor in our lives.

FOOD FOR THOUGHT

God loves you so much that he sent Jesus for you—so take great encouragement in the plans he has for you.

COURAGE TO FOLLOW

When Jesus heard this, he said to him, "You still lack one thing. Sell everything you have and give to the poor, and you will have treasure in heaven. Then come, follow me." When he heard this, he became very sad, because he was very wealthy. —Luke 18:22–23

Jesus doesn't ask everyone to sell all of his or her possessions in order to follow him. But he does call all of us to change in significant ways. These moments when we're called to change test our faith and courage. Do we really trust Jesus enough to give up familiar ways and try something new?

It's easy to change things we want to change, but God often asks for what we're holding on to the tightest. If we're clutching our possessions too closely, he may ask us to give them away. If fatigue is keeping us from loving others well, he may ask us to give up our frantic pace of life. If certain foods are our source of comfort, he may ask us to change the way we eat.

We have everything to gain by stepping out in trust. What is Jesus asking you to change today?

FOOD FOR THOUGHT

If we dare to follow Jesus and change, we will have everything to gain.

PATIENT TRUST

Say to the Israelites: "I am the LORD, and I will bring you out from under the yoke of the Egyptians."
　　　　　　　　　　　　　　　　　　　　　　　　—Exodus 6:6

God told Moses to confront the Egyptian pharaoh and demand that he let the Israelites leave Egypt. Pharaoh responded by making the Israelites' forced labor even more difficult. Moses complained that God had made things worse for his people. God responded by promising he would free his people.

Sometimes God takes time to transform our lives. He doesn't do it all at once, because he wants us to persevere in trusting him. Sometimes things even look worse for a while before they get better. Then, when freedom finally comes, we are filled with gratitude and deeper trust instead of taking God's provision for granted.

What are you trusting the Lord to do for you? When he seems to be taking too long, or even seems silent, don't give up. Keep crying out to him for help. He kept his promise to Moses, and he'll keep his promises to you.

FOOD FOR THOUGHT

Believe God, trust his timing, and be grateful for his deliverance when it comes. It will come.

EMBRACING THE NEW

Ruth replied, "Don't urge me to leave you or to turn back from you. Where you go I will go, and where you stay I will stay. Your people will be my people and your God my God. Where you die I will die, and there I will be buried. May the LORD deal with me, be it ever so severely, if even death separates you and me." —Ruth 1:16–17

Ruth could have stayed in Moab, but she chose to leave everything familiar to her and join Naomi, who was sunk in grief after losing her husband and two sons. Naomi needed her, and Ruth chose faithfulness to her mother-in-law over familiarity and security. She even chose Naomi's God, the Lord, over the gods of Moab.

Ruth had the courage to embrace change. She had suffered a severe loss, the death of her husband, but she didn't let grief immobilize her. Her resilience gave her what she needed to put herself in a position where the Lord could bless her circumstances and use her to bless others. We, too, need that resilience, that courage to accept change. God gives us grace in those moments and carries us when we need it most. What courageous step is the Lord asking of you today?

FOOD FOR THOUGHT

God can bring good out of any circumstances, even in unfamiliar territory.

NOTHING DEEPER THAN HIS LOVE

Know this love that surpasses knowledge—that you may be filled to the measure of all the fullness of God. —*Ephesians 3:19*

God's love is deep enough to handle anything. No matter what hurt you have experienced in the past, what problems you're going through right now, or what pain you will face in the future, you can count on God's love. There may be days when you feel you have hit bottom and could not possibly go any lower. Well, beneath what feels like the bottom is the bedrock of God's love.

That bedrock is solid enough for you to build a changed life upon. There's no need to tiptoe forward, worrying about mistakes. God embraces you in the messiness of the change process. He is thrilled that you've begun the process, and he is present every moment to give you strength when you ask for it.

FOOD FOR THOUGHT

God's love for you is deeper than any pain or mistakes, and he is with you right now.

MARVELOUS WORK

How you made me is amazing and wonderful. I praise you for that. What
you have done is wonderful. I know that very well.

—*Psalm 139:14 NIrV*

God has made your body with strengths and weaknesses unlike those of anyone else. You'll get a lot further with your healthy choices if you take the time to understand the way you were made. For instance, maybe you have brittle bones—those will affect the kinds of exercise and supplements you need. Maybe you have a slower metabolism, so you need different portions of food to flourish. Maybe your knees can handle running, or maybe they can't, and you'd be better off swimming. It may be tempting to bemoan all the things that seem like flaws to you, but God wants you to thank him for making you so wonderfully complex.

Genuinely thank God for the way your body is made, focusing on the things you can do and accepting the things that look like flaws to you. God loves you with all of those features.

FOOD FOR THOUGHT

You are uniquely made with strengths and weaknesses, both of which can be used to glorify God.

LOVE FROM THE DEEP

God knows how much I love you and long for you with the tender compassion of Christ Jesus.
—*Philippians 1:8 NLT*

The Greek word translated as "tender compassion" here means guts or intestines. The Greeks believed human emotions came from the internal organs of the belly. Paul is telling the Philippians he loves them from his gut, the way Jesus loves them.

This is the kind of love we need to have for our friends. The support of someone who loves us the way Jesus does can make all the difference in hardship, in resilience, and in transformation. We need love from them, and they need it from us. Mother Teresa said, "Love is a fruit in season at all times and within reach of every hand."

We don't drum up supernatural love by trying harder. Instead, we pray for it. Elsewhere Paul says God "has given us the Holy Spirit to fill our hearts with his love" (Romans 5:5 NLT). As we offer ourselves to be filled with the Holy Spirit, we will also be filled with his love.

FOOD FOR THOUGHT

If we ask him, God will fill us with a supernatural love for others.

AKA ENCOURAGER

Then Barnabas went to Tarsus to look for Saul, and when he found him,
he brought him to Antioch. So for a whole year Barnabas and Saul met
with the church and taught great numbers of people.

—Acts 11:25–26

A believer named Joseph got the nickname "Barnabas," which meant "Son of Encouragement" (Acts 4:36), because he had a habit of encouraging others.

Many believers were suspicious of a new convert named Saul, who had formerly tried to get the authorities to arrest the followers of Christ. But Barnabas staked his reputation on standing up for Saul as an honest and repentant convert, and others accepted Saul because Barnabas did. Later, Barnabas saw Saul's remarkable teaching gifts and asked Saul to join him in ministry in Antioch. Barnabas made it his business to see to it that Saul reached his full potential. His encouragement paid off: Saul was later known as the apostle Paul, one of the foremost leaders of the church.

Our friends need us to be sons and daughters of encouragement. They need us to notice and point out their gifts and strengths. They need us to root for them when their courage falters and they get off track. Who can you encourage this week?

FOOD FOR THOUGHT

One encouraging friend can be so life giving that it affects our progress and our success.

PERSISTENT PRAYER

In her deep anguish Hannah prayed to the LORD, weeping bitterly.

—*1 Samuel 1:10*

In a culture where a woman's worth was measured by the number of her sons, childless Hannah was scorned. Her husband had a second wife with several children, and that second wife made Hannah miserable. So when the family journeyed to the place where God's tabernacle was set up for worship, Hannah poured out her heart in prayer.

God heard that persistent and impassioned prayer, and he gave her a son. He grew up to be a leader of Israel as both priest and prophet. When Hannah dedicated him to the Lord's service as a small boy, she prayed another prayer (1 Samuel 2:1–10) on behalf of the entire nation, praising God not just for his goodness to her, but also for his goodness to all of Israel.

God hears persistent, passionate prayer. Persistence honors our relationship with him. What will you bring to him?

FOOD FOR THOUGHT

God honors our prayers and carries our anguish close to his heart.

BOUNDLESS POTENTIAL

"Can we find anyone like this man, one in whom is the spirit of God?"
—*Genesis 41:38*

We can't judge our potential by our circumstances. God may be shaping us to do something powerful in his service. For example, Joseph spent much of his young adulthood as a slave in Egypt after his jealous brothers sold him to some slave traders. If he had judged his potential by those circumstances, he would have been discouraged indeed.

But God had plans for Joseph. He used a chance meeting in prison to propel Joseph into the service of Egypt's pharaoh. Pharaoh recognized the spirit of God in Joseph, and Joseph became the number two man in the nation. He devoted his talents to planning for a famine that would have killed tens of thousands in Egypt and the surrounding nations. God used him to save countless lives, including those of the family who had sold him.

God has purposes for your life that you may not see yet. Don't underestimate what he can do with someone whose life is yielded to his service.

FOOD FOR THOUGHT

You have the Holy Spirit in you, and he gives you boundless potential for good in the world.

FINDING CONTENTMENT

I have learned to be content whatever the circumstances. I know what it is to be in need, and I know what it is to have plenty. I have learned the secret of being content in any and every situation, whether well fed or hungry, whether living in plenty or in want. —Philippians 4:11–12

The apostle Paul sat in prison, chained to a guard, waiting for possible execution, but he didn't let his circumstances sap his courage. In fact, he told his friends in Philippi, he had learned the secret of contentment. That secret was a rock-solid certainty that his life was worth living if he could be of use to God, and that was far more important than being comfortable.

None of us wants to be hungry or without basic necessities, and we can rightly pray for relief. Yet we can, like Paul, also find contentment with whatever our circumstances are. Contentment comes from passionate commitment to God's higher purposes.

FOOD FOR THOUGHT

Contentment is a great blessing, because it makes joy and peace possible regardless of circumstances.

GOOD INTENTIONS

Joseph said to them, "Don't be afraid. Am I in the place of God? You intended to harm me, but God intended it for good to accomplish what is now being done, the saving of many lives. —Genesis 50:19–20*

When Joseph rose to become the chief minister of Egypt's pharaoh, he had the opportunity to take revenge on his brothers for selling him into slavery years earlier. Instead, he forgave them. He gave two reasons for choosing forgiveness.

First, he said, "Am I in the place of God?" To withhold forgiveness is to claim the place of judge that only God deserves. We are in no position to demand punishment for others when we want mercy for ourselves.

Second, he saw God's hand in the events, turning even cruelty to good. By selling him as a slave, his brothers had placed Joseph in the right place at the right time to limit the harm of a famine that swept through the Middle East.

Our friends and family will inevitably fail us sometimes, and we desperately need the humility and confidence in God that enabled Joseph to choose forgiveness over bitterness.

FOOD FOR THOUGHT

Forgiveness is possible and can transform your life with the freedom only God can provide.

THE GOOD RISK

*Jesus said, "Daughter, you took a risk trusting me, and now you're healed
and whole. Live well, live blessed!"*　　　　　　　*—Luke 8:48 MSG*

Awoman with a chronic illness was convinced that if she touched
even Jesus' clothes, she would become well. But the Law of Moses
declared that bleeding made a woman ritually unclean, so she would
make anyone she touched also unclean. Still, she crept up to Jesus and
touched his clothes in secret.

He, however, didn't want her healing to be secret. He insisted
that she step forward and identify herself. She dared to do that, and
Jesus praised her for taking the risk.

He wants us to take that same risk, reaching out to him without
fear of being shamed. He doesn't see us as unclean, and nothing in us
defiles him. If we take the risk of opening ourselves up fully to God
and asking for what we need, our spiritual healing is guaranteed.

What healing do you need from Jesus? He will rejoice as you put
your wholehearted trust in him.

FOOD FOR THOUGHT

The risk of trusting God is always worth it; he will
always respond to meet our deepest need.

RELATIONAL GLUE

Be kind and compassionate to one another, forgiving each other, just as in Christ God forgave you. —Ephesians 4:32

The glue that holds healthy relationships together is kindness, compassion, and forgiveness. We all make mistakes and fall short, so we all need to give *and* receive forgiveness on a regular basis. Billy Graham said, "Every human being is under construction from conception to death."[16]

Since we have received enormous forgiveness from God, it's only fair that we treat others the same way. Likewise, we have received compassion and kindness from God. He is compassionate and gentle, suffering with us when we suffer. That's what our friends need from us: not necessarily fixing the problem, but the gift of our comforting presence.

We instinctively know how to be kind to a child who skins his knee: we hug and listen, and when the hurt has passed, we coax the child to get up and play again. The same compassion is appropriate when a friend suffers a loss or faces a trial. Even adults need physical touch and a listening ear.

FOOD FOR THOUGHT

Kindness, compassion, and forgiveness lead to strong relationships that will sustain us through the ups and downs of life.

SOLID FOOTING

The Sovereign LORD *is my strength; he makes my feet like the feet of a deer, he enables me to tread on the heights.* —*Habakkuk 3:19*

The prophet Daniel possessed strength beyond the size of his muscles—he had strength of faith, courage, obedience, devotion, dedication, endurance, and discipline. Because of him we speak about being Daniel Strong, which is a pursuit of excellence in body, mind, and spirit for God's glory. We could just as well speak of being Habakkuk Strong, because this prophet, too, found his strength in God. Habakkuk lived in a time of economic and political instability, so he needed stability from God to carry him through the challenges of an uncertain future.

Whatever challenges you face, God wants to give you solid footing so your faith stays strong. He wants to be your daily source of strength beyond the size of your muscles. He can empower you. As the Bible says, "The LORD is my strength and my shield; my heart trusts in him, and he helps me" (Psalm 28:7).

FOOD FOR THOUGHT

Being Daniel Strong is all about strength in body, mind, and spirit.

HIS HAND

Because the hand of the LORD my God was on me, I took courage and
gathered leaders from Israel to go up with me. —Ezra 7:28

E zra was a priest in exile in Babylon, but God convinced him to
lead a contingent of his fellow Jews back to Israel. It was a dangerous journey, hundreds of miles to walk, with enemies along the way
and enemies when they arrived. But God's hand was on Ezra's goal:
to help the people of Israel resettle in their land and follow the law of
God. Thousands of Jews had gone back to Israel years earlier, and they
needed someone like Ezra who was gifted in teaching. So Ezra took
courage and set off on the journey of a lifetime to serve God according
to his gifts.

Fulfilling our goals to the glory of God takes courage. We need
the hand of the Lord on us. Ezra relied on prayer for protection against
enemies, and we, too, need to rely on prayer to deal with obstacles we
face. Ezra said, "We fasted and petitioned our God about this, and he
answered our prayer" (Ezra 8:23).

FOOD FOR THOUGHT

The hand of the Lord is on you when you pursue
goals for his glory; have the courage to take another
step forward into new territory.

FEARLESS

For I am the LORD your God who takes hold of your right hand and says
to you, Do not fear; I will help you. —Isaiah 41:13

Ask yourself, "If I could realize or accomplish anything related to my health and fitness, without fear of failure, what would it be?" Let yourself dream as big as you can. Do you want to get your blood sugar under control, feel enthusiastic and energetic when you get out of bed in the morning, lift your mood, manage stress, complete a 5K, get a peaceful night's sleep, learn to swim, or spend an active day with your grandkids without getting exhausted?

Whatever your dream is, when it aligns with God's purposes, God takes hold of your hand and says he will help you. He can make your dream possible if you give it to him. He says, "Who always gets things started? I did. GOD. I'm first on the scene. I'm also the last to leave" (Isaiah 41:4 MSG). So put your dreams in God's hands. He will be with you every step of the way.

FOOD FOR THOUGHT

God will help you accomplish your goals and dreams in ways that bring honor to him.

NOURISHED

Why do you spend your money on junk food, your hard-earned cash on cotton candy? Listen to me, listen well: Eat only the best, fill yourself with only the finest. Pay attention, come close now, listen carefully to my life-giving, life-nourishing words. —Isaiah 55:2–3 MSG

We know the health benefits of eating real food grown on a plant rather than manufactured in a plant. Real food is medicine; junk food is toxic. God says the same is true in the spiritual realm: his Word is real food for our souls. It renews our minds and replenishes our spirits. We need it in our daily diet. Consider making a plan to read a portion of one of the Gospels, one of Paul's letters, or a psalm each morning or before you go to bed.

God invites us to partake of spiritual food that will make our souls flourish. "God's Word is better than a diamond, better than a diamond set between emeralds. You'll like it better than strawberries in spring, better than red, ripe strawberries" (Psalm 19:10 MSG).

How can you feed your soul and body today?

FOOD FOR THOUGHT

God's words are truly life-giving and life-nourishing, real food for the hungry soul.

THE PAYOFF

Easy come, easy go, but steady diligence pays off.

—*Proverbs 13:11 MSG*

We often take for granted the things that come to us easily. Diligence is persistent effort for things that do not come easily, and it's one of the main virtues we need in our pursuit of a healthy lifestyle.

For instance, getting enough movement in a busy day takes diligence to schedule time to walk or lift weights. Meal plans take diligence because we have to plan ahead for grocery shopping, chopping vegetables, and cooking. Along with improving our health, all this diligence provides a bonus in the rest of our lives. It can help us to be more faithful in relationships, so that people increasingly know they can depend on us. It can help us become more consistent in time with God. It can help us with financial decisions. Diligence is a muscle well worth exercising, because it has benefits far beyond our physical health.

FOOD FOR THOUGHT

A practice of diligence pays off in every area of life.

PROPELLED BY JOY

Surely God is my salvation; I will trust and not be afraid. The LORD, the LORD himself, is my strength and my defense; he has become my salvation.
—*Isaiah 12:2*

Scott Kretchmar, professor of Exercise and Sports Science at Penn State says, "When movement is experienced as joy, it adorns our lives, makes our days go better, and gives us something to look forward to. When movement is joyful and meaningful, it may even inspire us to do things we never thought possible." God wants to take you on a journey toward experiencing movement as joy. He wants to lead you to a place where you revel in what your muscles can do, where every time you lift or bend or stride you can say, "Give praise to the LORD, proclaim his name; make known among the nations what he has done" (Isaiah 12:4)!

When you get to a place where movement is joyful for you, you'll be amazed at what you'll be inspired to do. Let his joy propel you there.

FOOD FOR THOUGHT

You *can* get to a place where you experience movement as joy and offer it to God as praise.

WHO YOU ARE

"You're blessed when you're content with just who you are—no more, no less. That's the moment you find yourselves proud owners of everything that can't be bought."　　　　　　　　*—Matthew 5:5 MSG*

It's good to have goals that stretch us, as long as we know that reaching those goals isn't the measure of our worth. We need a spirit of contentment that says, "I'm loved and secure just the way I am. I don't need to be more or less to please other people. God treasures me the way I am, even if I don't reach my goals, even if I have good days and bad days." This secure, loved place is the stable foundation for pursuing goals, because contentment frees us from the fear of failing. We move forward toward our goals with peace instead of anxiety.

The Bible says, "Godliness with contentment is great gain. For we brought nothing into the world, and we can take nothing out of it" (1 Timothy 6:6–7). How content are you with who you are right now?

FOOD FOR THOUGHT

You're blessed with peace if you're content with who you are right now.

IN SADNESS

Be joyful with those who are joyful. Be sad with those who are sad.
—Romans 12:15 NIrV

We live in a world where loss and failure happen to everyone. We can lose health, jobs, friends, finances. We need the skills to deal with losses rather than papering them over with "happy" talk. Jesus was "a man of suffering and familiar with pain" (Isaiah 53:3), and we need to be like him in dealing authentically with grief.

Community is essential to grieving well. When our friends suffer a loss, we need to be there with them. Otherwise, the loss can be too big to bear. The first thing we can do as friends is to provide a listening ear and a caring heart. Our friends need a place to say, "It was bad. It really hurts."

Henri Nouwen said, "The friend who can be silent with us in a moment of despair or confusion, who can stay with us in an hour of grief and bereavement, who can tolerate not knowing . . . not healing, not curing . . . that is a friend who cares."[17]

Do you know anyone who has suffered a loss? Offer a listening ear and your loving presence.

FOOD FOR THOUGHT

We give our friends a tremendous gift when we're available to listen and mourn with them.

HEAVENLY GRAIN

He rained down manna for the people to eat, he gave them the grain of heaven. Human beings ate the bread of angels; he sent them all the food they could eat. —Psalm 78:24–25

When the Israelites wandered in the desert for forty years before entering the Promised Land, God fed them with miraculous food called manna. It tasted like wafers made with honey, and it appeared each morning, six days a week, like frost on the ground. On the sixth day there was enough for two days, and on the Sabbath they rested and gathered no manna. God provided for them in this just-enough-for-today miracle so they would learn that "man does not live on bread alone but on every word that comes from the mouth of the LORD" (Deuteronomy 8:3). They needed to understand how utterly dependent they were on God and how generous he was in providing for them.

God provides for us, too, sometimes just enough for today. We have a much broader abundance of food choices than just manna day after day—that's something to be grateful for! When we eat and are satisfied with the goodness of real food, let's celebrate the generosity of the God who gives it to us.

FOOD FOR THOUGHT

In his abundant generosity, God gives us all the food we need to nourish us completely.

HELD IN LOVE

But God demonstrates his own love for us in this: While we were still sinners, Christ died for us.
—Romans 5:8

The greatest motivation to change is love. We need to know how deeply God loves us, because then we'll be able to take small steps of change without fear of failure. God loves you so much that he sent his Son to die for you. That's not just a nice notion; it's a truth you can bank on. He sacrificed what was most dear to him to express his undying love for you. If he's done that, won't he also come through for you again when you need help? Yes, he will.

There will never be a moment in this life when God is not paying attention to you. The psalmist recognized this about God: "If I settle on the far side of the sea, even there your hand will guide me, your right hand will hold me fast" (Psalm 139:9–10). God is guiding you, holding your hand as you take steps to improve your health. No matter what each day holds, reflect on the profound truth that Christ died for you, and God's presence is near you.

FOOD FOR THOUGHT

You can risk change because God's love for you is endless; he is always ready to guide you.

EXEMPLARY FRIEND

You are the children that God dearly loves. So follow his example. Lead
a life of love, just as Christ did. He loved us. He gave himself up for us.
He was a sweet-smelling offering and sacrifice to God.
—Ephesians 5:1–2 NIrV

If we want to know how to treat our friends, we can simply look to the way God has treated us. Christ sacrificed his very life on our behalf. While we won't be called upon to die for our friends, we will have opportunities to sacrifice our own agenda when a friend is in need. We'll sacrifice time and energy to listen to a friend and do practical acts of service.

Often we're so busy with our assigned work and home life that relationships get our leftover energy, if we have any. However, Christ invites us to carve out time to care for each other. This may mean simply slowing down and sacrificing our time, money, or assistance to a co-worker or family member who needs more than our productivity.

How can you walk in the way of love today?

FOOD FOR THOUGHT

We have the privilege of doing for others what God has done for us: love sacrificially.

GOD-PLEASER

Without faith it is impossible to please God.

—Hebrews 11:6

It will take faith to achieve and maintain the total health that God desires for you. Part of that faith is the conviction that life is about trusting God's unlimited power instead of your limited willpower. People of faith are those who admit they can't do it on their own. Humility is an essential ingredient of their lives.

You've already begun to embrace your powerlessness and God's strength. Continue to trust him, surrendering all of your goals and desires to him and asking him to bring to fruition what he has planned for you.

Perfect performance isn't what pleases God. What warms his heart is total surrender and faith in his power and his promises. Author and theologian Brennan Manning said, "to live by grace means to acknowledge my whole life story, the light side and the dark. In admitting my shadow side, I learn who I am and what God's grace really means."[18]

What do you need faith for today?

FOOD FOR THOUGHT

Pleasing God is as simple as trusting him as your Savior and Lord, letting him guide your steps.

CONSTANT TALK

Never stop praying.

—*1 Thessalonians 5:17 NIrV*

It's good to develop morning and evening rituals when you draw near to God and set aside time to focus on him. You can be nourished and refreshed by his presence and ask for the grace to follow through with all he has called you to. If things have gone well, you can celebrate with God. If things haven't gone as well, you can ask for the power and faith to get back on track. Enter his presence with eagerness to receive his affection and encouragement, as his love for you is unconditional and never based on your performance.

God longs to communicate with you. He knows what's on your heart without being told, but he wants to have the kind of relationship with you where you confide in him. He also wants to speak to you through his Word, through other people, and through thoughts when you are at prayer. The more you turn your thoughts to him in the morning, in the evening, and throughout the day, the more he will be able to replenish your heart with his love.

FOOD FOR THOUGHT

God is always present, waiting for an ongoing conversation with you.

CONNECTIONS OF PEACE

If it is possible, as far as it depends on you, live at peace with everyone.
—Romans 12:18

The health of our relationships influences our physical health. For example, sometimes we eat because we're lonely or unhappy in a relationship. Stress often comes from relationships and gets expressed in our bodies as headaches, high blood pressure, sleeplessness, or muscle tension. And on the positive side, when our relationships are deep and satisfying, we have energy freed up to give to physical activities. We feel alive, eager to move, and eager to serve God.

These are some good reasons to seek peace in relationships. Seeking peace means doing what we can to resolve conflict in constructive ways, talking honestly and respectfully about differences. It means making the other person's needs a priority alongside our own needs. It means offering forgiveness and asking for forgiveness.

Are any of your relationships causing you stress? How can you seek peace in those relationships? "Blessed are the peacemakers, for they will be called children of God" (Matthew 5:9).

FOOD FOR THOUGHT

God will bless you, and your body will thank you, if you do your part to make peace with the people around you.

STEADY, STEADY

God himself is right alongside to keep you steady and on track until things are all wrapped up by Jesus. —1 Corinthians 1:8 MSG

Imagine this: God himself is right next to you right now. His hands are ready to steady you. He will keep you on track with your health and faith, proving that you can continue to trust him as your savior and manager of your life. He will keep you on track with your food and fitness if you ask him to. He will keep you on track in your relationships and your mental focus. All you have to do is stay connected with him moment by moment.

And what happens if you stray off track? He is still right there. No blame, no condemnation. He calls you to make a U-turn and get back on course. Those course corrections are part of how he trains you so that you learn what works and what doesn't. Over time staying on track will start to feel normal. Imagine that.

FOOD FOR THOUGHT

Right now, God is alongside you, keeping you moving steadily toward the goals he has planned for you.

RECEIVING MERCY

Anyone who hides their sins doesn't succeed. But anyone who admits their sins and gives them up finds mercy. —Proverbs 28:13 NIrV

God promises mercy to those who confess and turn from their sins. But what do we tend to do instead? Hide or ignore it? Brush it off? Justify it?

Hiding sins and setbacks from God and others only makes it more likely that we'll continue in the same destructive pattern. It also drains our energy, because our conscience keeps trying to tell us that something is wrong. We create a reservoir of guilt and shame that we can only keep secret with effort. The psalmist says that when he kept silent about his sin, "My bones wasted away through my groaning all day long" (Psalm 32:3).

But when we confess the mistakes we've made, God washes away the guilt and shame. God doesn't condemn us; he welcomes us into his embrace and gives us a chance to start fresh. He also gives us the strength to choose and act differently next time. All it takes is the humility to be honest about what happened.

FOOD FOR THOUGHT

U-turns are not only allowed in God's kingdom; they're encouraged. He offers mercy without limit.

RUNNING TEAM

Do you not know that in a race all the runners run, but only one gets the prize? Run in such a way as to get the prize. Everyone who competes in the games goes into strict training. They do it to get a crown that will not last, but we do it to get a crown that will last forever.

—1 Corinthians 9:24–25

The apostle Paul encourages us to train hard to win the gold medal of God's eternal blessing. In an ordinary race, he says, only one person wins. Everyone is competing against everyone else. In the Christian life, though, because we are all on the same team, we run alongside each other. We complement others' strides, while they complement ours.

There's a proverb from Zambia that says, "When you run alone, you run fast. When you run together, you run far." If you're trying to build healthy habits for a lifetime, you're running a marathon, so you need your brothers and sisters spurring you on. There will be moments when you stumble, and at those times your fellow runners will help you regain your balance and renew your strength to persevere to win the prize.

Who are the people who are in the race with you, the ones who care whether you keep going or quit? Check in with one of them today.

FOOD FOR THOUGHT

When you run together, you run far, finishing the race and rejoicing together.

GOD'S GUARANTEE

For we know how dearly God loves us, because he has given us the Holy Spirit to fill our hearts with his love.   —Romans 5:5 NLT

Your body is a temple of the Holy Spirit. He lives inside you (1 Corinthians 6:19), filling your heart with his love. The Holy Spirit in you is God's guarantee that his love will never leave you. Whenever you need help to move forward in your healthy lifestyle, you can call on the Holy Spirit, and he is there with power and with reassurance of God's love.

Human love is conditional. People say, "I love you if . . ." or "I love you because . . . ," and when circumstances change, their love fades. But God's love is unconditional, so he will never, never stop loving you. Your sins and failures don't stop him from loving you. This is the secure place from which you can dare to make changes and deal with mistakes. As author and theologian Brennan Manning said, "Define yourself radically as one beloved by God. This is the true self; every other identity is illusion."[19]

FOOD FOR THOUGHT

The Holy Spirit in you is God's guarantee that his love for you is unconditional and permanent.

HEALTHY ENOUGH TO LOVE

You made me and formed me with your own hands. Give me understanding so that I can learn your commands. —Psalm 119:73 NIrV

Why does God care whether you eat right, get enough exercise, and get enough rest? Because he wants you to have enough energy to love him, love your family and friends, and even love people you don't know well. Loving God and others is your main reason for being on this earth (Matthew 22:37–40), and it's hard to love when you're exhausted. Love takes patience, and patience is so much easier when you are full. Love takes vitality, and real food is medicine that makes your body feel better. Imagine having the energy to ride a bicycle with your grandchildren or help a friend move to a new house. You might even write down loving things you want to be able to do when you're healthier.

So if you're looking for a motivation that will sustain you as you make healthy changes in your life, consider making love your aim.

FOOD FOR THOUGHT

Love is a terrific motivation for making healthy changes, because love is ultimately what will make you feel most alive and joyful.

SURRENDERING WHAT YOU LOVE

*God said, "Take your son, your only son, whom you love—Isaac—and go
to the region of Moriah. Sacrifice him there as a burnt offering..."*
—Genesis 22:2

As a test of faith, God told Abraham to sacrifice his beloved son.
When Abraham obeyed, God stopped him just before he struck
Isaac with the knife. This situation is unimaginable—what a picture
of complete faith! The Bible says Abraham trusted that God was even
able to raise Isaac from the dead (Hebrews 11:19).

Sometimes God asks us to give up something or someone we
love. It may be something that isn't good for us. It may be something
good in itself, but God wants us to let go of it. He calls us to do that by
faith, trusting that he has his reasons and he is able even to raise the
dead in his own time. These are hard moments, and we often don't
understand why they come. But there is a blessing for choosing faith
over doubt. God is always wise, always good, always trustworthy,
even when we don't understand why he asks us to let go of something
we're attached to.

FOOD FOR THOUGHT

Sometimes, offering our "Isaac" to the Lord is essential on the road to full surrender and peace.

THE SOVEREIGN GOD

*Yours, LORD, is the greatness and the power and the glory and the majesty
and the splendor, for everything in heaven and earth is yours.*

—*1 Chronicles 29:11*

God is sovereign. This means he rules over every event, no matter how small, and he is in control of what happens to us. He knows everything—nothing is a mystery to him. He has perfect wisdom. He knows the outcome of anything anyone does. He has all power; he can do anything that is consistent with his nature. By his sovereignty, he rules all of creation.

Because God is sovereign, we can have lasting change and spiritual growth only if we cooperate with God to pursue them. We can't change on our own, yet he won't change us without our cooperation. In his love, he has granted us the freedom to choose whether and how we want to change. We have the awesome privilege of partnering with the Creator of the universe in shaping our lives according to his design.

FOOD FOR THOUGHT

Pursue your transformation, knowing that the sovereign God is working in you according to the plan he dreamed for you when he created you.

THE SHORTEST PATH TO GOD

I will give thanks to you, LORD, with all my heart; I will tell of all your wonderful deeds. —Psalm 9:1

Brennan Manning said, "The dominant characteristic of an authentic spiritual life is the gratitude that flows from trust—not only for all the gifts that I receive from God, but gratitude for all the suffering. Because in that purifying experience, suffering has often been the shortest path to intimacy with God."[20]

Suffering may not seem like a path to intimacy with God. But we find ourselves driven to seek God more when we are suffering than when everything is fine. And when we need him desperately, we find he is more than enough. We find ourselves sharing in the sufferings of the crucified Christ (Philippians 3:10) and thus understanding his sacrifice in a way that we couldn't learn any other way. He endured terrible suffering and still stayed close to God, and in our suffering we can have a glimpse of how it is possible for us to do the same.

FOOD FOR THOUGHT

Suffering gives us the priceless gift of drawing closer to God and discovering that he is more than enough.

MAX FAITH

Make every effort to add to your faith goodness; and to goodness,
knowledge; and to knowledge, self-control; and to self-control, perseverance.
—2 Peter 1:5–6

Faith is foundational. By itself, though, faith can do only so much. That's why Peter urges us to add other character qualities that bring faith to its fullest potential. These additional qualities include goodness, knowledge, self-control, and perseverance.

These qualities can be easily translated to our health journey. As we learn the best foods to eat, we can then ask God to help us develop the self-control and perseverance to make those foods a steady part of our diet. We can grow in self-control by planning ahead and being intentional about what we eat. By planning ahead, we'll always have good choices available to nourish us. By being mindful in this way, and doing it consistently, we use our knowledge, self-control, and perseverance. Then our bodies will be at their best for whatever service the Lord asks of us.

FOOD FOR THOUGHT

Adding an array of virtues to our faith will transform us to be increasingly like Jesus.

BIG DIVIDENDS

You can develop a healthy, robust community that lives right with God and enjoy its results only if you do the hard work of getting along with each other, treating each other with dignity and honor.

—*James 3:18 MSG*

A few high-quality relationships will take you farther along the road toward health than a mass of casual acquaintances. You need people who will love you at your worst—when you've been eating all the wrong foods, when you've been too busy to work out, when you're mad at yourself for getting off track. These are the people whose patience will help you rise above your bad days and whose acceptance will help you begin again.

Relationships like that don't happen automatically. As James says, we need to do the hard work of getting along with each other. We take time for each other, listening closely. We talk about the real issues in our lives, below the surface of saying everything is "fine."

Who are the people in your life who might become supportive friends? What step can you take this week to do the hard work of better developing those relationships?

FOOD FOR THOUGHT

The hard work of getting along with true friends pays big dividends in support of our health goals and our life.

ALWAYS THERE

Those who know your name trust in you, for you, LORD, have never forsaken those who seek you.   —*Psalm 9:10*

On the twists and turns of your journey toward health, God will never forsake you. You may have days when stress gets the better of you and you make all the choices you didn't want to make, but those days don't discourage God. He is always ready to offer a fresh start.

It's worth asking God, "What got me off course? What was the trigger that started it all? What could I do differently next time?" Ask these questions in a spirit of curiosity, not self-blame. Aim to treat a rough day as a source of useful information and contemplation.

The Bible says, "You, LORD, hear the desire of the afflicted; you encourage them, and you listen to their cry" (Psalm 10:17). That's God's stance toward you: hearing your cry, understanding the challenge, listening and encouraging. He wants to be your encourager and steadfast source.

FOOD FOR THOUGHT

God never forsakes us. He listens, he encourages, and he extends his hand to help us.

TUNING IN

Let your ears listen to wisdom. Apply your heart to understanding.
—Proverbs 2:2 NIrV

Making healthy choices is easier when you grow in wisdom. Wisdom is practical understanding about how to live well.

One area of wisdom on the journey toward healthier living is learning the skill of choosing the best foods and mastering the practice of reading food labels. A wise person discerns the potentially misleading marketing claims like "natural" or "healthy" and instead goes straight to the list of ingredients in small print. If you don't know what any of the ingredients are, stay away from that food. For instance, maltose, dextrose, maltodextrin, and evaporated cane juice are all types of sugar. You don't have to memorize all the types of chemicals and processed ingredients to build wisdom, just use common sense to look for real food and stay away from ingredients you don't know.

Wisdom grows with practice. Reading labels is a skill that becomes easier—even second nature—with practice. It takes time to tune your ears and eyes, but it's worth it.

FOOD FOR THOUGHT

Wisdom is key to living a long and healthy life.

UNSTOPPABLE COURAGE

When they saw the courage of Peter and John and realized that they were unschooled, ordinary men, they were astonished and they took note that these men had been with Jesus.

—*Acts 4:13*

When Jesus was arrested, Peter was afraid to be identified as one of his followers for fear that he, too, would be arrested. But after Jesus rose from the dead, the Holy Spirit filled Peter on the day of Pentecost, and from then on, Peter was fearless. He stood up to the ruling council in Jerusalem, the same council that had condemned Jesus. The councilors were astounded at the courage of Peter and John. Peter had not just been with Jesus physically; he had been with Jesus on a transformative journey of experiencing his life, death, and resurrection.

Peter's goal was to lead as many people as possible to surrender their lives in service to Jesus Christ. He was giving to others from the abundance that he had received. And it was his experience of being with Jesus that gave him courage. Being with Jesus can give you courage like Peter's to pursue your call for the glory of God.

FOOD FOR THOUGHT

Being with Jesus can give you unstoppable courage to pursue his dreams for you.

THE LORD IS PEACE

So Gideon built an altar to the LORD there and called it The LORD Is Peace.
—Judges 6:24

One of God's names in the Bible is *Yahweh-Shalom*, which means the Lord is Peace. The Hebrew word for peace, *shalom*, means wholeness in all of life, completeness, welfare, safety. God is our source of all of these blessings.

Philosopher Cornelius Plantinga explains shalom like this: "In the Bible, shalom means universal flourishing, wholeness and delight—a rich state of affairs in which natural needs are satisfied and natural gifts fruitfully employed, a state of affairs that inspires joyful wonder as its Creator and Savior opens doors and welcomes the creatures in whom he delights."[21]

That's what we long for in our journey toward physical and spiritual health: flourishing, wholeness, and delight. Picture the doors flung open and our Prince of Peace (Isaiah 9:6) welcoming us into a place.

FOOD FOR THOUGHT

The Prince of Peace welcomes us to a place of flourishing, wholeness, and delight.

LIVING GOD'S WAY

But what happens when we live God's way?.... We develop a willingness to stick with things.... We find ourselves involved in loyal commitments, not needing to force our way in life, able to marshal and direct our energies wisely.
—Galatians 5:22 MSG

Living God's way, empowered by his Holy Spirit, leads us to become increasingly willing to persevere. It also helps us develop patience and self-control, which are invaluable for developing a healthier lifestyle.

Consider exercise, for instance. If you ask God for help, the Holy Spirit will enable you to be more willing to stick with movement you enjoy. If you need help to stick with a healthy eating plan, the Spirit will provide that help. Once you ask, then go into your activity or your meal plan expecting God to empower you with perseverance and self-control. Choosing to live God's way and depending on his Holy Spirit will enable you to do it.

FOOD FOR THOUGHT

God will help you develop the willingness to stick with the things that lead to a life full of health and energy.

INCALCULABLE VALUE

By his power God raised the Lord from the dead, and he will raise us also.
—1 Corinthians 6:14

If you are a follower of Jesus Christ, God is going to raise your body from the dead when Jesus comes back. This means your body matters to God as much as your soul does right now. God designed you to have a body, and it is of immense value to him.

No earthly parent would say that she cares about her child's soul but not his body. She counts the child's fingers and toes, and treasures every feature of his face. Your heavenly Father loves you more than any earthly parent, and he cherishes every part of your body.

Your current body is also like a church, a holy house for the Holy Spirit. "Do you not know that your bodies are temples of the Holy Spirit, who is in you, whom you have received from God?" (1 Corinthians 6:19). How are you moved to take care of your body today?

FOOD FOR THOUGHT

Your future resurrection with a body means your body now is valuable to God.

SPIRITUAL VITAMINS

Do not be wise in your own eyes; fear the LORD and shun evil. This will bring health to your body and nourishment to your bones.

—*Proverbs 3:7–8*

One of the best things you can do for your physical health is to stay spiritually healthy. Proverbs 3:7 speaks of just two of the many aspects of spiritual health that matter to God: humility and integrity.

First, "Do not be wise in your own eyes." In other words, don't think you know all that you need to know. Even if you know a lot of information, information isn't the same as wisdom. Be open to wisdom from God. Wisdom comes from taking God seriously and yourself less seriously. It comes from walking with God day after day, learning his ways.

Second, "Fear the LORD and shun evil." Have a healthy awe of God's power and justice so that you live with integrity. Expect that choosing to do what is right will be richly rewarded.

How can you pursue wisdom today? What step of integrity can you take?

FOOD FOR THOUGHT

Humility and integrity are like vitamins, nourishing both body and soul.

FEARLESS LOVE

Perfect love expels all fear. If we are afraid, it is for fear of punishment, and this shows that we have not fully experienced his perfect love.

—*1 John 4:18 NLT*

Fear and love don't get along well. If we are afraid of someone, it's hard to love him or her. That's true in our relationship with God, and it's true in our relationships with other people. If we're afraid of being hurt or used, we shy away from getting close to people.

God wants to help us move into relationships fearlessly. He wants to help us gradually become so secure in his love that we can deal with another person's flaws.

We need to let people get close. We need to let them know the real us, the best and the worst, so that they can support us. If we fear rejection, we can pause before we go into an interaction and ask God for help. We can say, "God, please give me the courage to take a step toward this person." That's a prayer he's eager to answer.

FOOD FOR THOUGHT

When we're confident of God's perfect love, we can move into relationships fearlessly.

WAITING EXPECTANTLY

In the morning, LORD, you hear my voice; in the morning I lay my requests before you and wait expectantly.　　　　　　　　　　—Psalm 5:3

Just as a morning routine of a good breakfast is healthy for the body, so a morning routine of prayer and Bible reading is nourishing for the spirit. It's like a daily Sabbath when we take time away from our responsibilities to sit at the Lord's feet. We lay our requests before him and wait expectantly for him to answer. Sometimes all we need is the reminder of his gracious presence surrounding us.

The Bible says, "Your word, LORD, is eternal; it stands firm in the heavens" (Psalm 119:89). No matter what else is going on in our lives, God's Word is sure. The Bible also says, "I will walk about in freedom, for I have sought out your precepts" (Psalm 119:45). True freedom comes from seeking out, absorbing, and living by God's ways. Daily time with even a small portion of God's Word connects us to him for the day.

FOOD FOR THOUGHT

When we wait expectantly for the Creator of the universe each morning, he draws near to us and restores our souls.

RIGHT THERE

Whoever dwells in the shelter of the Most High will rest in the shadow of the Almighty. I will say of the LORD, "He is my refuge and my fortress, my God, in whom I trust." —Psalm 91:1–2

We never have to be lonely, because God is always present with us. To dwell in his shelter is to maintain conscious connection with him throughout the day. We can maintain it by offering short prayers, such as the name of Jesus or "You are my refuge" or "I trust you, Lord." We can also schedule short breaks in the day to meditate on him—his goodness, his love, his faithfulness.

The psalmist says to God, "I am always with you; you hold me by my right hand. You guide me with your counsel, and afterward you will take me into glory" (Psalm 73:23–24). God is always, always there, close enough to hold us by the hand, eager to guide us, promising to take us into glory. How amazing it is that right now you are with him.

FOOD FOR THOUGHT

God is our refuge and fortress, the Friend who always stands with us, and he longs for us to seek his presence.

FRIENDS WHEN IT COUNTS

Therefore confess your sins to each other and pray for each other so that you may be healed. —James 5:16

When we're having a rough day or make an unhealthy choice, sometimes the best thing we can do is contact a friend. We don't have to deal with the struggle alone. And sometimes what we really need is God working through one of his people.

The Bible says, "A friend loves at all times, and a brother is born for a time of adversity" (Proverbs 17:17). Times of adversity are when we most need someone else in our corner. Just knowing another person is thinking of us and will pray for us can boost our hope.

The best kind of friend when we're lonely, frustrated, or defeated is someone we can be honest with. Who is one person who can handle hearing about your sin or your mistakes? Who is one person who will pray and not judge you? That's a friend who will help you on the road to healthy living.

FOOD FOR THOUGHT

Treasure the friends who can deal with hearing about your weaknesses. They will help you heal.

THE PRAYER INITIATIVE

We never stop praying for you. . . . We pray that he will make you worthy of his choice. We pray he will make every good thing you want to do come true. We pray that he will do this by his power. We pray that he will make perfect all that you have done by faith. —2 Thessalonians 1:11 NIrV

Imagine someone praying for you all the time, praying that God will make you fit for what he's called you to be. Imagine someone praying that God will fill your good ideas with his own energy so that what you do amounts to something. Your truly supportive friends can pray that way for you, and you can pray that way for them. Ask God to help them know, believe, and fulfill what he is calling them to be.

In any relationship, somebody needs to take the initiative to keep the relationship going. Prayer is one initiative that will build up your friendships. Consider committing to praying 2 Thessalonians 1:11 for a friend, family member, or someone in your small group. And let them know you're praying for them.

FOOD FOR THOUGHT

God longs to fill your acts of faith with his own energy so that every act bears rich fruit in your own and others' lives.

FIT TODAY AND FOREVER

*Workouts in the gymnasium are useful, but a disciplined life in God is far
more so, making you fit both today and forever.*

—1 Timothy 4:8 MSG

Picture yourself Daniel Strong—physically, emotionally, relationally, and spiritually fit. What would your body look like? Who are
the people you would be standing with? What are your relationships
like? What would spiritual fitness enable you to do?

The way to get there is to set goals for yourself. Goals are the steps
we take each day, week, and month to get from where we are today to
the future we dream of having. Goals are part of the disciplined life
the Bible speaks of. What steps can you take each day that will add up
to a disciplined life?

God wants you to be all that he's created you to be. He's right
alongside you, empowering and encouraging you. What are the small
steps of discipline that he's inviting you to take today?

FOOD FOR THOUGHT

A disciplined life in God will make you physically,
emotionally, relationally, and spiritually fit, fulfilling
your desires and enabling you to walk the path God
desires for you.

WITH YOU

*The angel of the LORD encamps around those who fear him, and he
delivers them.*
—*Psalm 34:7*

The king of Aram once sent an army against the prophet Elisha because Elisha was helping Israel defend itself in a war with Aram. One day, Elisha and his servant woke up to find their town surrounded by armed men. Elisha's servant panicked, but Elisha said, "Don't be afraid . . . Those who are with us are more than those who are with them" (2 Kings 6:16). His servant didn't know what he was talking about—he saw only the two of them alone—until Elisha asked the Lord to open his servant's eyes. Then he saw an army of angels encamped in the surrounding hills.

If you need courage to do something God has given you to do, remember that those who are on your side are more than those who are against you. You may not see God's angels, but they are there to deliver you. What brave thing is he calling you to do today?

FOOD FOR THOUGHT

Move forward with bold confidence knowing that God's angels surround you.

RELYING ON GOD

We were under great pressure, far beyond our ability to endure, so that we despaired of life itself. Indeed, we felt we had received the sentence of death. But this happened that we might not rely on ourselves but on God, who raises the dead. —2 Corinthians 1:8–9

The apostle Paul and his missionary team were often in life-threatening danger. On one occasion he wrote to the believers in Corinth about his situation. He said he was pushed beyond his own resources and faced death. But the experience taught him to rely on God, who raises the dead.

There's really no way to learn to rely on God other than to be pushed beyond our own resources. That's one of the reasons God allows those situations. If you feel overwhelmed by some circumstance, consider letting it propel you into God's arms. Also, ask your Daniel Plan friends to pray for you. That's what Paul did, and he looked forward to the thanksgiving his friends would offer up when he was delivered from danger (2 Corinthians 1:11). He also knew that the experience would someday help him comfort others under similar pressure (2 Corinthians 4–5). God never wastes pain or hardship.

FOOD FOR THOUGHT

God is in your current circumstances and committed to bringing good out of them.

SATISFIED

The poor will eat and be satisfied; those who seek the Lord will praise him.
—*Psalm 22:26*

D r. Mark Hyman says, "Food has the power to heal us. It is the most potent tool we have to prevent and treat many of our chronic diseases." The reason to eat real food is not to fit into our jeans or to look good in a dress or to be a certain size for a family reunion, but it's to be awake to the beauty and miracle of life. The reason is to be able to live with purpose, to love, to serve, to connect, to celebrate all the gifts God has given us. What we put on the end of the fork has the power to equip us with the energy and vitality to live for God.

Dr. Hyman also says, "The beauty of adding food that heals, nourishes, and satisfies you deeply is that it will almost effortlessly shift your body and mind into a state where you naturally crave what makes you thrive and feel good." It's time to thrive.

FOOD FOR THOUGHT

Real whole food has the power to give us the energy we were designed to live with.

NEVER LET DOWN

So let God work his will in you. . . . Say a quiet yes to God and he'll be there in no time.　　　　　　　　　　　　　　　　　　　—*James 4:7–8 MSG*

As we're on The Daniel Plan and trying to move forward in five essential areas of health, we are bound to face temptations to quit. We are bound to face setbacks and relapses. That's part of growing—three steps forward and two steps back. There is no straight line toward our goals. When the steps back happen, we don't need to be discouraged. God will never let us down, and he'll never let us be pushed past what we can endure. He will move in close and offer help if we let him.

Instead of focusing on the two steps back, celebrate the three steps forward. Progress is what matters, not perfection. Over time, there will gradually be more forward steps than setbacks, leading to big results in the long run.

FOOD FOR THOUGHT

Amid setbacks and temptation, God is at your side. He's helping you up and moving you on your way again toward victory.

WORD REVIVAL

I lie in the dust; revive me by your word.

—Psalm 119:25 NLT

When stress has flattened us, God's Word can be like a nutrient-packed drink providing the energy we need to get on our feet again. The stories of God's intervention in the lives of biblical men and women (Moses, Gideon, Hannah, Zacchaeus, etc.) can remind us that he is working for good in his people's lives. As the psalmist says, "The law of the Lord is perfect, refreshing the soul.... The precepts of the Lord are right, giving joy to the heart. The commands of the Lord are radiant, giving light to the eyes" (Psalm 19:7–8).

God's promises, too, can uplift our souls. There are thousands of them, and we can count on every one. For instance, "When you pass through the waters, I will be with you; and when you pass through the rivers, they will not sweep over you" (Isaiah 43:2). Stress may be like rough waters, but God promises he will enable us to swim safely to shore.

FOOD FOR THOUGHT

God's Word is a treasure trove of nourishment for the stressed-out soul.

WAY TO THRIVE

These are the proverbs of Solomon. . . . They provide you with instruction and help you live wisely. They lead to what is right and honest and fair.
—Proverbs 1:1, 3 NIrV

Discipline is about creating habits. When we create small habits, together they build into big results. These habits might be sleeping a bit more, moving our bodies, calming our minds, eating a little differently, adding a few new foods that are positive, refocusing our thoughts and replacing them with God's Word. Any habits that help us toward health will increase our capacity for self-care and healing.

One of the most fruitful habits we can form in the areas of food and fitness is to add joy to the way we move and the way we eat. When we experience movement as joy, we celebrate the fact that our bodies were designed for motion. Movement can become an offering to the God who made our bodies. Likewise, taking joy in trying food that nourishes us or trying a new food can celebrate the abundance God has provided. Each day, we can look forward to practicing new habits and enjoying the pleasures God has in store for us.

FOOD FOR THOUGHT

Small habits lead to ever greater enjoyment of the life God has blessed us with.

DOING THINGS WE NEVER THOUGHT POSSIBLE

No discipline is enjoyable while it is happening—it's painful! But afterward there will be a peaceful harvest of right living for those who are trained in this way.
—Hebrews 12:11 NLT

At first, discipline comes with pain. Our muscles are sore when we start a new activity or raise the challenge to a new level. We're tired. We may even experience cravings for our old ways of eating or living as change takes us into unfamiliar territory.

Over time, though, the discipline becomes a habit. We become accustomed to movement and the slight soreness of exercised muscles. It's a good feeling to increase the weight or the duration as our strength builds. We feel a sense of accomplishment. The cravings soon fade away. The unfamiliar becomes familiar and we feel peaceful because we know we're living well.

So when the discipline is painful, we can keep going if we fix our eyes on the peaceful harvest ahead. God will be with us in the process, helping us to do what we never thought possible.

FOOD FOR THOUGHT

Fix your eyes on the peaceful harvest ahead that comes with diligent training.

WE'RE WEAK

*I will boast all the more gladly about my weaknesses, so that Christ's power
may rest on me.*   —2 Corinthians 12:9

When a problem can't be fixed, it can be endured. Not only can
we survive it, but we can also use it to grow more like Christ.
The apostle Paul faced many kinds of opposition that he couldn't stop.
He had to endure them, not in his own strength but in God's. God told
him, "My grace is sufficient for you, for my power is made perfect in
weakness" (2 Corinthians 12:9). So Paul reveled in his weaknesses
because they pointed him to God's grace. Just as he cried out to God
for help, we too can do the same.

We don't have to handle problems on our own. As soon as we turn
to God and pray for his strength and wisdom, he is right there enabling us to bear it. He "gives grace to the humble" (James 4:6 NKJV).
Humility means admitting we're human and need God. What a relief
it is to accept that.

FOOD FOR THOUGHT

Not only can we survive with weaknesses, we can
thrive if we are depending on God for his power to
work through our weakness.

MAKE ROOM FOR PEOPLE

Carry one another's heavy loads. If you do, you will fulfill the law of Christ.
—*Galatians 6:2 NIrV*

When problems overwhelm us, God's grace comes to us in many forms. Sometimes he empowers us directly. Sometimes he guides us through his Word. And sometimes he works through other people. He wants us to accept their encouragement and practical help. Will you be humble enough to ask for help from his people?

He never meant for us to go through life on our own. That's why the Bible speaks of God's people as limbs of one body: Christ's body. "The eye cannot say to the hand, 'I don't need you!' And the head cannot say to the feet, 'I don't need you!'" (1 Corinthians 12:21). We all need each other to face what life dishes out. If you're in over your head or just feeling lonely, ask someone for help or a listening ear.

FOOD FOR THOUGHT

Accepting help from others honors them and enables them to fulfill the design God created for them.

INVESTIGATION

We take captive every thought to make it obedient to Christ.
—2 Corinthians 10:5

Dr. Daniel Amen says, "Thoughts exert a powerful influence over your life and body. Uninvestigated thoughts provide the emotional fuel for anger, anxiety, depression, and unhealthy behaviors." Mental health requires that we investigate our thoughts, asking ourselves whether they are true in reality and line up with what Scripture teaches.

God will show us what is true and help us reframe our thinking. For instance, we may need to shift our thinking so that we believe it is possible for us to move forward in faith, food, fitness, focus, and friends. We may need to believe that God will give us the power to grow. We can believe King David when he says, "It is God who arms me with strength and keeps my way secure" (Psalm 18:32) and "The Lord gives strength to his people; the Lord blesses his people with peace" (Psalm 29:11). As we examine our thinking through God's perspective, we will increasingly live in ways that honor God.

FOOD FOR THOUGHT

Take the time to investigate your thoughts in light of God's truth.

LIFE-GIVING ENERGY

How abundant are the good things that you have stored up for those who fear you.
                                                              —Psalm 31:19

As you start to eat real food, your cravings and addictions will be replaced by deep pleasure and satisfaction from naturally sweet things, such as a variety of delicious fruits, including dates, berries, pears, as well as vegetables like red bell peppers and sweet potatoes. Dr. Mark Hyman says, "The power of real food creates an abundant, healthy life. You can get the most powerful life-giving energy from your food."

Health starts in the kitchen. The best thing we can do for our health is to focus on all the amazing foods God has given us: fresh fruits, fresh vegetables, nuts, and seeds.

Food is information. It has the ability to change our genes. It can reverse chronic conditions and give us the vitality we were created to have. Once you start to enjoy real food, you'll never want to settle for less. God has given us an amazing array of foods to nourish and replenish us. What amazing choice will you try today?

FOOD FOR THOUGHT

Don't settle for anything less than God's best, especially with food.

ENTERING GOD'S REST

Come to me, all you who are weary and burdened, and I will give you rest.
Take my yoke upon you and learn from me, for I am gentle and humble in
heart, and you will find rest for your souls. —Matthew 11:28–29

Jesus gives us an incredible promise of entering into God's rest, of finding rest for our souls as we draw near to him. But how can we draw near unless we carve out time to enter his loving embrace?

Rest isn't only for our souls; it's also for our minds and bodies. In our limited capacity on earth, we can only go so long before we need a break. But if we regularly rest, then we allow God to replenish us long before we've overextended ourselves.

Fitness expert Sean Foy says one of the best things we can do for our bodies, especially if we are challenging ourselves on a regular basis, is to take a break. This is one of the best things we can do for our souls as well. Take a break. Carve out time for quiet in your life. Make it a habit.

FOOD FOR THOUGHT

Being intentional about respite is invaluable for our minds, bodies, and souls.

DEARLY LOVED

Follow God's example, therefore, as dearly loved children and walk in the way of love, just as Christ loved us and gave himself up for us as a fragrant offering and sacrifice to God. —Ephesians 5:1–2

The more deeply we believe that we are God's dearly loved children, the more able we will be to walk in the way of love. Christ loved us so much that he gave himself up for us. We need to ponder that so we can see our identity as the Beloved.

Henri Nouwen said, "Every time you feel hurt, offended, or rejected, you have to dare to say to yourself: 'These feelings, strong as they may be, are not telling me the truth about myself. The truth, even though I cannot feel it right now, is that I am the chosen child of God, precious in God's eyes, called the Beloved from all eternity, and held safe in an everlasting embrace.'"[22]

If we truly believe the truth that we are the Beloved, we will find it more and more natural to treat others with love and live the way we were designed to live.

FOOD FOR THOUGHT

We are dearly loved children of the best Father there can be. Nothing can separate us from his love.

STABLE HOPE

When doubts filled my mind, your comfort gave me renewed hope and cheer.
—Psalm 94:19 NLT

What doubts visit you often? Doubt fills our minds from time to time, especially when circumstances get overwhelming. In the early stages of practicing The Daniel Plan, we may be influenced by doubts about whether changing what we eat will really change the way we feel. We may doubt whether we have the strength to move more. Doubts come from our past experiences, from naysayers, and from ideas deeply rooted in our culture.

When those doubts come up, let's take them to God and ask him for clarity about what is true. Let's ask him to bring wise people into our lives, people we can trust. If we doubt our abilities, we can look at God's unlimited abilities and find renewed hope.

If you have doubts, focus on a truth from God's Word. Hope in him; nothing is more stable or comforting.

FOOD FOR THOUGHT

Even when we have doubts, God can give us renewed hope and joy to keep moving forward.

GOD CARES

Cast all your anxiety on him because he cares for you.

—1 Peter 5:7

Anxiety begins with worrisome thoughts—and they influence our bodies. Anxiety can affect our breathing, heart rate, hormones, and other biological functions. The way to counteract anxiety is to breathe slowly and deeply. On each out-breath, think about or repeat a truth from God's Word. Next, tell God each anxious thought, each situation that causes worry or fear. Slow down, breathe and then say the truth, which is that God cares for you and has your circumstances completely under his control.

Pray or meditate on biblical truths such as Psalm 31:7, "I will be glad and rejoice in your love, for you saw my affliction and knew the anguish of my soul." Or Psalm 34:4, "I sought the LORD, and he answered me; he delivered me from all my fears."

Is there anything troubling you today? Offer it up to God. He'll affirm the truth of his love for you.

FOOD FOR THOUGHT

God cares for us as his own children, so we can entrust all our concerns to his wisdom and love.

LIGHT IN THE DARKNESS

I will instruct you and teach you in the way you should go; I will counsel you with my loving eye on you. —*Psalm 32:8*

When we're not sure what to do, God offers to give us counsel. If we truly desire to follow him, he will provide us with direction. The main way he does this is through his Word. The Bible says, "Your word is a lamp to guide my feet and a light for my path," (Psalm 119:105 NLT). In the darkest circumstances, his Word shines as a light to show us where to step. When we're in a dark place, the Word can encourage us about which way to go and what dangers to avoid. His wisdom takes us from fumbling around in the dark to taking clear, confident steps in the daylight. We have every reason to want his light to mark our way every day.

God really is with us, providing the practical wisdom we need to make good decisions in each area of life.

FOOD FOR THOUGHT

How blessed we are to have the bright light of God's Word shining on our path, showing us the way to move forward into the future God designed for us.

SEEKING HIM

Search for the LORD and for his strength; continually seek him.
—1 Chronicles 16:11 NLT

In order to have what it takes to become Daniel Strong, we need to continually seek the Lord and his strength. We can seek him in his Word and in prayer; we can also search for him in the circumstances of our lives and the people around us. Let's ask him to open our eyes to all the places where he is at work. Look for the Lord with the same curiosity and enthusiasm that a child has when searching on an Easter egg hunt.

God is hiding in plain sight. Where is he at work in your family? How can you cooperate? Where is he active in your workplace, in your children's school, among your friends, in your eating plan? Every time you find him present in another person or place, you'll gain more strength to do what pleases him.

Search for him like treasure, and he will reward you with the strength you need.

FOOD FOR THOUGHT

The Lord rewards those who seek him continually, providing them with the faith, love, strength, and wisdom they need to have lives that bless themselves and other people.

NEW EYES TO SEE

Be content with what you have, because God has said, "Never will I leave you; never will I forsake you."
                                                                    —*Hebrews 13:5*

Being content and being grateful go hand in hand. A contented heart is one that can see all the blessings, rather than focus on what's missing. Sometimes we aren't grateful for something until it is taken away. We appreciate our health once we've been sick. We appreciate our friends when we lose one, or the roof over our heads when we need to move. How much better, though, to stand back and ask God to give us new eyes to see clearly the good things in our lives before we lose them. We take an active role in being grateful, in choosing to see the goodness God has provided. There may be some shadows in the painting of our lives, but those, too, are worthy of thanks because they allow us to see where God's light is.

Contentment grows when we develop an intentional habit of being thankful for the small things that happen every day. Contentment grows when we ask God to give us new eyes to see the good we are experiencing. Take an inventory of your blessings today.

FOOD FOR THOUGHT

Contentment makes our lives far richer because it allows us to see God's hand in every single thing.

HIDDEN DIAMONDS

True godliness with contentment is itself great wealth.

—1 Timothy 6:6 NLT

The preacher Russell Conwell told a story about a man who made a decent living from his land but sold the property to go in search of diamonds. He spent years in his search and eventually died hopeless and penniless. Meanwhile, the person who bought his property happened to find a beautiful rough stone in the sands of his streambed and put it on his mantel. A friend saw it there and told him it was a diamond. So they went out and dug in the sands and found acres of diamonds. They mined the land, and it became one of the most productive diamond mines in the world.

Too often we are blind to the riches on our own property. Contentment is great wealth because it teaches us to notice and be grateful for the rough and glittering stones at our feet, which may very well be uncut diamonds, if only we have eyes to see them. There may be such richness beneath the surface if we're willing to do a little digging.

What are the diamonds in your life that you may have overlooked?

FOOD FOR THOUGHT

We are unimaginably wealthy with all of the good things God has showered on us.

A BIG INVESTMENT

God chose us to belong to Christ before the world was created. He chose us to be holy and without blame in his eyes. He loved us. So he decided long ago to adopt us. He adopted us as his children with all the rights children have. He did it because of what Jesus Christ has done.

—Ephesians 1:4–5 NIrV

Even before he made the world, God knew just what you would be like—how he would design you and the choices you would make—and regardless of anything you've done, he knew you and loved you.

God invested in you first by creating you, second by sending his Son to die for you, and third by inviting you to be part of his family. What an unimaginable investment, the price of Christ's suffering and death! Picture Jesus with his arms outstretched on the cross saying, "I love you this much."

If God has invested so much in you, wouldn't it make sense to invest in the care of your body and soul? How can you take care of yourself today?

FOOD FOR THOUGHT

God has invested so much in us, and we have the privilege of investing and caring for the bodies and souls he gave us.

THE ONE WHO PROVIDES

Abraham called that place The LORD Will Provide. And to this day it is said, "On the mountain of the LORD it will be provided."

—*Genesis 22:14*

God always provided for Abraham, even at times when Abraham's faith was weak. During a famine, Abraham doubted God and went to Egypt, but even there, God provided for his family. Later, Abraham doubted that God would provide a son for him, and he took matters into his own hands, but God straightened out the resulting mess and gave Abraham a son with his wife, Sarah. By the time of the events of Genesis 22, Abraham was so accustomed to God's provision that he didn't question it.

God really is the King of kings and the Lord of lords. He's the creator of the universe. He doesn't treat us like slaves, but like sons and daughters, his very own, his beloved ones. We are his family, and he delights in providing for us abundantly just as any parent does. Genesis 22 even gives "provider" as one of his names: Yahweh-yireh, or the Lord Will Provide. As we make changes in our lives, we can have the security of knowing that he can provide for every need.

What needs will you put into his hands today?

FOOD FOR THOUGHT

God builds our faith when we let him be in charge and provide for us.

CELEBRATING SMALL CHANGES

You, LORD, are our Father. We are the clay, you are the potter; we are all the work of your hand.
—Isaiah 64:8

Sometimes it can be easy to get caught up in looking at how far we are from being a finished piece of pottery instead of celebrating what a beautiful work of art God has already made. We focus too much on the weight we haven't lost, the sleep we haven't had, and the amount of time we sit instead of moving.

Instead, we need to celebrate the small changes: the one pound lost, the one healthy lunch, the one supportive friend, the body that *did* move today. And remember the big wins that depend solely on God: his grace and mercy for our sins, the new life he gives us in Christ, the Holy Spirit living in us.

God's plan to mold and shape us takes time to unfold. There are no shortcuts. It all happens in God's time. To be patient in the waiting, we can remind ourselves that "He who began a good work in you will carry it on to completion" (Philippians 1:6).

How are you already a work of art? What small changes can you celebrate?

FOOD FOR THOUGHT

You are clay in the loving potter's hand, and he will sculpt and mold you until completion.

SET APART FOR GOD'S PLAN

"Before I formed you in the womb I knew you, before you were born I set you apart."
—Jeremiah 1:5

God had a plan for you before your mom even knew you would be born. He set you apart as his chosen instrument. What if you viewed yourself this way? What if you could see the way God is leading you to transform your health in body, mind, and soul? What if you knew that you could be so much healthier now than you were ten years ago? Jesus said, "With man this is impossible, but with God all things are possible" (Matthew 19:26).

God's plan for you is based on who he made you to be and who he wants you to become. It's based on his ideas. It's uniquely tailored for you by the one who knows you better than anyone else. He will make you more and more like Christ and will shape you to complete your mission. And this *uniquely you* plan is powered by his mighty power that formed the universe and raised Christ from the dead.

FOOD FOR THOUGHT

You can accomplish things you never thought possible as you embrace God's unique design for your life.

ON YOUR SIDE

"Do not be afraid; do not be discouraged, for the Lord your God will be with you wherever you go."
           —Joshua 1:9

God gave Joshua the daunting task of leading his people into the Promised Land. They would have to drive out the wicked inhabitants, so they had many years of warfare ahead of them. They didn't have superior weapons or skills; what they had was the promise that the Lord would be with them and he would fight for them.

God makes that same promise to you: He will be with you wherever you go when you seek to honor him with your life and be transformed into the likeness of his Son. He will be with you as you choose to love him with all your heart, soul, mind, and strength. He will be with you as you love others as he has loved you. He asks you to be strong *in* him and courageous *because* of him, wherever he leads you.

FOOD FOR THOUGHT

You can be strong and courageous, because God will be with you wherever you go, giving you the power to do what he has prepared for you.

STEPPING OUT

If the LORD is pleased with us, he will lead us into that land, a land flowing with milk and honey, and will give it to us. —Numbers 14:8

Twelve Israelites went into the Promised Land to survey it and bring back intelligence to the people. All twelve agreed that it was good land, but ten of the men said it would be impossible for the Israelites to conquer it. Only two—Joshua and Caleb—said that God would enable the Israelites to take the land.

Eyes of fear focus on difficulties and underestimate your abilities. Eyes of faith look to God and see his sufficiency. Which kind of eyes do you have? Maybe God is asking you to take a step of faith on your journey to improve your health. Perhaps he wants you to try the ten-day detox or the forty-day meal plan. Maybe he's asking you to try a new kind of movement or a new mindset, and instead it feels like you're facing powerful enemies. But if God really is asking you to take that step of faith, he will be the one to carry you forward.

FOOD FOR THOUGHT

God is all the courage you need to step out in faith toward all the goals and dreams you have.

HOPE IN GOD

And so, Lord, where do I put my hope? My only hope is in you.
—*Psalm 39:7 NLT*

Hope is a simple but confident expectation from a God who is so much bigger than we can imagine. Faith gives us the power to hold on to hope whether it rains or shines. When everything seems dark, hope is the light that comes through the crack in the door. The Bible says, "The Lord is good to those whose hope is in him, to the one who seeks him; it is good to wait quietly for the salvation of the Lord. . . . there may be yet hope" (Lamentations 3:25–29).

Do you need hope? Consider going off alone in silence, bowing, and waiting for the Lord. There's nothing you need to say unless you want to say it. Just be with God and let him show you the light coming through the crack in the door.

FOOD FOR THOUGHT

When we passionately wait for and diligently seek God, he will fill us with confident expectation that he will come through.

DEFEATING DISTRACTIONS

Many are the plans in a person's heart, but it is the LORD's purpose that prevails.
—Proverbs 19:21

D r. Daniel Amen says, "In a world where there are so many distractions competing for our attention, it is more important than ever to focus on God's plan, promises, and priorities for your life." We need time each day when the television and social media are turned off so that we can think deeply about what God has in mind for us.

According to media strategist Melissa Leiter, the lifespan of a Twitter tweet can be as brief as a couple of seconds. A Facebook post might remain in a newsfeed for two hours. By contrast, God's words have lasted for centuries and will keep on lasting. His plans are eternal. He has known you from the foundation of the world, and his purposes for you are unchanging and profoundly good.

Take some time today to tune out the fleeting messages the world is sending you so that you can think about what's eternal. This will put into perspective the short-term plans that crowd your heart, and then you'll be able to hear and agree with the Lord's purposes for you.

FOOD FOR THOUGHT

Screening out the distractions that clamor for your attention will give you a clear mind to focus on what really matters.

WITH GRATITUDE

Enter his gates with thanksgiving and his courts with praise; give thanks to him and praise his name.
—Psalm 100:4

Life is always less than perfect, so there's always something to complain about if we want to. But the Bible says, "Do everything without grumbling or arguing" (Philippians 2:14). Why? Because the negativity snowballs if we entertain it. On the other hand, if we focus on the things we have to be grateful for, we enter God's gates with thanksgiving.

In The Daniel Plan we encourage you to write down at least three things you're grateful for every day. Writing them down for even a couple of weeks can measurably increase your level of happiness and contentment.

It's also helpful to tell someone what you're grateful for, especially if it's something they have done. Saying thank you uplifts both of you. And if there's a concrete way you can show your gratitude, like doing something for someone else or giving a gift, that will root you even deeper into the fertile soil of contentment.

FOOD FOR THOUGHT

If we meditate on what we're grateful for, we will supercharge our moods and have a far richer experience of God's powerful presence.

PURE AND SIMPLE

But I am afraid that . . . your minds may somehow be led astray from your sincere and pure devotion to Christ. —2 Corinthians 11:3

God calls us to a pure and simple devotion. Often our lives can become too complicated, and we may need to let go of some of the baggage that weighs us down, both in our spiritual lives and our journey toward health. We need to eliminate detours like envy, bitterness, jealousy, and comparison with others. We need to simplify our schedules so that we can live with vitality, enjoying God and life-giving movement. We need a simple eating plan with pure foods. We need simplified goals to focus on.

What are the distractions that get in the way of your pure and simple devotion? What leads you away from putting God first and then building on that with food, fitness, focus, and friends? How can you declutter your life so that you maintain pure and simple devotion to God and your health?

FOOD FOR THOUGHT

Pure and simple devotion to Christ enables us to focus on what truly matters and move forward with our life-giving goals.

THURSDAY

DEATH-DEFYING POWER

"Not by might nor by power, but by my Spirit," says the LORD *Almighty.*
—*Zechariah 4:6*

We will not succeed in The Daniel Plan by sheer effort, but by the strength of the Holy Spirit. God's power is made perfect in our weakness (2 Corinthians 12:9). He wants us to rely solely on the power he provides, the same power by which he raised Jesus Christ from the dead. That death-defying power is available daily. God wants to give us lives full of energy and momentum as we plug into his power source.

When we face an uphill battle, we must yield our hearts and minds to the sustaining grace of a loving God. And at those moments when his power seems to elude us and his grace seems far away, we seize the opportunity to practice patience and cling to the promises in his Word. The psalmist cries out to God, "I lie in the dust; revive me by your word" (Psalm 119:25 NLT). He doesn't pretend to lead a self-sufficient life. He completely surrenders and depends on God.

FOOD FOR THOUGHT

When we run to God, he gives the power of his Holy Spirit so we may accomplish his will.

THE WILLING HEART

"God goes against the willful proud; God gives grace to the willing humble."
—James 4:6 MSG

Willfulness is the stance that we don't need anybody other than ourselves to accomplish our goals. Will-lessness is the stance that our goals are impossible and it's not worth trying to meet them. God can do nothing for either the willful or the will-less person, the arrogant or the passive person. But in contrast to these is the willing person. This is the person of humble faith who says, "I can't do this on my own, but I'm willing to try if God gives me the strength." God gives grace to the willing person.

You may have moments when you want to throw in the towel on your Daniel Plan goals. Maybe you have had a setback or you are facing an overwhelming situation or transition. The important thing is to stay focused on Christ and keep going. Don't opt for will-lessness because the challenge is big. Stay willing so you are open to God's strength in every situation.

FOOD FOR THOUGHT

Humility is the key that unlocks the treasure chest of God's grace to do what would be impossible on our own.

ALIVE

I have been crucified with Christ and I no longer live, but Christ lives in me. The life I now live in the body, I live by faith in the Son of God, who loved me and gave himself for me. —Galatians 2:20

The life we're trying to live in The Daniel Plan is by faith in the Son of God. We have been put to death, and now Christ lives in us. This new life takes us where we could never go by ourselves. God transforms us by the life of Christ within us. We are energized and made fully alive by his presence in us.

The apostle Paul says, "For in him we live and move and have our being" and "We are his offspring" (Acts 17:28). This isn't try-harder Christianity. This is Christ-powered Christianity. We trust him to do the work through us. It's an intimate, loving partnership where we do the footwork of moving forward and he provides the power.

FOOD FOR THOUGHT

It always comes back to love. He loved us and gave himself for us, and therefore we can have new life in him.

SUNDAY

WISE INTENTION

Be very careful, then, how you live—not as unwise but as wise.
—Ephesians 5:15

Real change requires us to face the truth. The Daniel Plan will help us face the truth about ourselves, our relationship with God, our eating and exercise patterns, our purpose, and our relationships with those closest to us. If we're looking for a quick fix, we're not going to find it here, but if we want to build an authentically healthy life based on the truth of God and the sound advice of medical experts, then this is the place to be.

It's ultimately about being careful how we live, with choices that replenish our bodies, minds, and souls. The Daniel Plan builds our lives on a foundation of faith, and then it adds rejuvenating food, fitness, and thoughts—all with a community of friends so that we can maintain this new lifestyle for the long haul. We're going to make wise, intentional choices that lead to huge results in the long run.

FOOD FOR THOUGHT

Wise people make small, careful choices in a good direction that add up to a thriving life that honors God.

THE SAME FOR EVERYONE

You are tempted in the same way all other human beings are. God is faithful. He will not let you be tempted any more than you can take. But when you are tempted, God will give you a way out. Then you will be able to deal with it. —1 Corinthians 10:13 NIrV

Knowing that temptations are pretty much the same for everyone levels the playing field. We're all dealing with them—some in one area, others in another. And it's great news that God won't allow the temptation to be more than we can stand. He promises to show us a way to move beyond the temptation to solid ground. Through his Word and his Spirit, he always provides direction to keep us on track. His grace is so great that he doesn't just forgive our failures; he also gives us the power to turn around.

God will fit everything—our setbacks, our relapses, our failures—into his plan for our lives. He has the power to overcome it all.

FOOD FOR THOUGHT

God knows exactly what you're going through, and he provides a way past temptation.

LIVING BY FAITH

We live by faith, not by sight.

—2 Corinthians 5:7

Sometimes we hold on to things that we don't want to release into God's hands. It might be a possession or a habit or a relationship. We hold on because we can't imagine living without that thing, and we don't trust God to handle it properly. Yet he is a trustworthy God. If he takes something away, he will make sure we can live without it. He is a God of abundance, not deprivation. He invites us to entrust everything into his hands and to live by faith, not by sight, not by control.

God sees more than we ever could. Our vision is limited by time, but he sees the past and the future as well as the present moment. Our vision is limited by space, but he sees everything in the world, including the depths of every human heart. So let's trust the one who sees all, and not rely on our limited eyes and ears.

FOOD FOR THOUGHT

Living by faith means we're not weighed down with things we aren't meant to hold onto.

EYES AHEAD

We'd better get on with it. Strip down, start running—and never quit!
No extra spiritual fat, no parasitic sins. Keep your eyes on Jesus, who both
began and finished this race we're in. —Hebrews 12:1–2 MSG

Five times, the Bible compares becoming like Jesus to running a race. You're running this race right now, and your goal is to be conformed to his image (Romans 8:29), to be fully yourself, living the way he would live if he were in your shoes. If you're going to run well, you'll want to shed some baggage that weighs you down. That baggage may be a food habit or a negative thought pattern or an unhealthy relationship pattern that gets in your way.

Study Jesus and his life to see how he ran this race on earth. Watch how he dealt with people and with painful or frustrating circumstances. Watch how he related to the Father. He wasn't just God dressed up as a human; he took on the life of a man in every way except sin. Run with your eyes on Jesus, and you're sure to finish well.

FOOD FOR THOUGHT

When we lift our eyes and focus on Jesus in the race ahead, we run stronger.

CALL TO MIND

Remember the things I have done in the past. For I alone am God! I am God, and there is none like me.   —Isaiah 46:9 NLT

Remember. God wants us to call to mind who he is and what he has done. He wants us to take our eyes off our everyday circumstances to look up and look back. He wants to completely reshape our thoughts as we remember what he has done for us over the course of our lives. Recall those things, and be grateful for them. It's so easy to forget these past kindnesses and think only of current needs, but he wants us to remember.

Even more, he wants us to remember the things he did before we were born: calling Israel to be his chosen people and shaping a family into which the Savior could be born; sending Jesus to live on earth as a man like us; allowing Jesus to be killed for our sins; raising Jesus from the dead. When we call these mighty acts to mind, we are assured that he alone is God.

What do you need to remember today about God's deeds?

FOOD FOR THOUGHT

Remembering what God has done will remind us that God has more than enough goodness and power to help us reach our goals.

TRUSTWORTHY

The LORD is trustworthy in all he promises and faithful in all he does.
—Psalm 145:13

God has made thousands of promises, and he is trustworthy in every one of them. If you need the courage to take a step forward on your journey to improve your health with a meal plan or a new kind of movement or a way of thinking, then consider some of these promises:

"The LORD is good to all; he has compassion on all he has made" (Psalm 145:9).

"The LORD upholds all who fall and lifts up all who are bowed down" (Psalm 145:14).

"The LORD is near to all who call on him, to all who call on him in truth" (Psalm 145:18).

"He fulfills the desires of those who fear him; he hears their cry and saves them" (Psalm 145:19).

"The LORD watches over all who love him" (Psalm 145:20).

Those are just five trustworthy promises from one psalm! How thankful we can be that his Word is full of promises to nourish our faith.

FOOD FOR THOUGHT

God's promises are for you. Trust them because he is faithful.

JESUS IN CHARGE

He will be called Wonderful Counselor, Mighty God, Everlasting Father, Prince of Peace. —Isaiah 9:6

What do you call Jesus Christ? What you say about him influences the way you relate to him. Is he your Wonderful Counselor, the one who guides you in how to live your life? Is he your Mighty God, the one you turn to for strength? Is he your Everlasting Father, the head of your family who gives you your identity? Is he your Prince of Peace, your source of safety and wholeness? Can you say to him, "Mighty God, here I am. I'm yours. I want to have complete faith in you. Help me to see you for all you are."

Pastor Rick Warren says, "You take the wheel from here, Lord; you call the shots. Be the CEO of my life, become the chairman of the board. I'm putting a sign up that says I am under new management." Let Jesus be in charge of your life, managing your pursuit of a healthy lifestyle.

FOOD FOR THOUGHT

God longs for us to draw near to him and know him as Wonderful Counselor, Mighty God, Everlasting Father, and Prince of Peace.

WAITING PATIENTLY FOR GOD

*Be still before the L*ORD *and wait patiently for him.*

—*Psalm 37:7*

Being still before the Lord is the ultimate surrender. Gradually learn to set aside the many commitments of your busy life for a few minutes, surrender ever more deeply to him, and wait patiently for him. Wait first for him to make his presence known to you, and then wait for him to act in your areas of need.

In the journey toward a healthier life, it's sometimes hard to be patient. It's sometimes hard to explain the uncertainties and unexpected challenges God allows in our lives. Sometimes we look for explanations, yet God doesn't always clue us in. Waiting patiently means we embrace the mystery of God. He doesn't always tell us why things happen to us, but he promises we will always have the gift of his presence.

What are you waiting for God to do for you? Set aside an unhurried amount of time to be still before him, breathing deeply and contemplating his presence. Lay your needs before him, and rest in his goodness.

FOOD FOR THOUGHT

Abundant blessing awaits us when we surrender all our concerns and wait patiently in God's presence.

FAILING FORWARD

But as for me, I am poor and needy; come quickly to me, O God. You are
my help and my deliverer; LORD, do not delay. —Psalm 70:5

W hen the psalmist says he is poor and needy, he speaks for all of us. We all have areas of our lives where we're weak and in need of God's deliverance. And the wonderful news is that he desires to be our help and our deliverer.

When we misstep or even fail in reaching some goal, we don't need to be discouraged. God expects us to fail, not just once but repeatedly. He's never surprised when that happens. As long as we keep failing forward, keep picking ourselves up and moving on, we're right in the place God has for us. Three steps forward and two steps back is still progress, and we can learn from every setback.

FOOD FOR THOUGHT

God is the deliverer of all who know they are poor and needy, all who are willing to keep failing forward.

TRUST, DELIGHT, AND COMMIT

Trust in the LORD and do good.... Take delight in the LORD.... Commit your way to the LORD; trust in him and he will do this: He will make your righteous reward shine like the dawn. —Psalm 37:3–6

God will make the reward you receive for righteous choices shine like the dawn if you can do these simple things: Take time to yield to him in trust. Relax in his presence and delight in him. Ask him to take your trust even deeper as you commit your way to him. Whether you're facing some large challenge or you find aspects of The Daniel Plan daunting, this time with God can be so renewing for your heart and mind that you will find the courage to overcome your circumstances.

He understands that trust doesn't happen all at once, but Psalm 37 shows us a few ways to open our hearts, and to build and practice trust little by little each day.

Part of developing trust comes when you learn to enjoy his presence and goodness. Then your heart opens more and more to him. When your delight is truly in him and not in any earthly comforts, the Bible says, "he will give you the desires of your heart" (Psalm 37:4).

FOOD FOR THOUGHT

Trust, delight, and commit—three glorious steps toward a reward that shines like the dawn.

THE PASSWORD

Enter with the password: "Thank you!" Make yourselves at home, talking praise. Thank him. Worship him. For GOD is sheer beauty, all-generous in love, loyal always and ever. —*Psalm 100:4–5 MSG*

Gratitude draws us near to God. Praise for his beauty, love, and loyalty settles us in his house. We can't see his beauty directly, but we can see it in the beautiful and good things he has made. His generosity in love means that he showers us with it far beyond what we deserve or even imagine. His loyalty means that he will never withdraw his love for us. The apostle Paul says, "Give thanks in all circumstances; for this is God's will for you in Christ Jesus" (1 Thessalonians 5:18). The reason we can be thankful in all circumstances is that God himself doesn't change.

The God who made billions of stars as beautiful and powerful as our sun actually wants us to become comfortable with the generosity he lavishes on us. He wants us to awake every day to the wonder that he has made us, preserves us in safety, and provides for our needs. He wants us to marvel at his generous gift of Jesus as a sacrifice to rescue us from death.

The password to his heart is "Thank you."

FOOD FOR THOUGHT

A few minutes of saying thank you every day will give you a taste of God's beauty, all-generous love, and loyalty.

HE MAKES YOU GREAT

Your right hand sustains me; your help has made me great. You provide a broad path for my feet, so that my ankles do not give way.

—*Psalm 18:35–36*

In Psalm 18, David gives us a vivid picture of God meeting us where we are and providing what we need. David is a warrior, and he's grateful that God arms him with strength, makes his feet sure-footed, sustains him, and clears the path for him to march on. When he says, "your help has made me great," the word *help* could equally be translated as *gentleness* or *humility*. Imagine God humbling himself, bending down to our level so that he can give the help we need. Imagine him sweeping the rocks out of our path so that we don't turn an ankle as we step forward.

As we're trying to make changes on The Daniel Plan, we can easily feel stuck on what looks like a steep and rocky path. We may feel we've gone only one mile on a twenty-five-mile hike. Yet David says God will clear the path and be our support each and every mile.

FOOD FOR THOUGHT

Right now, God is bending down to clear and widen the path for you.

VIEW FROM ABOVE

He makes my feet like the feet of a deer; he causes me to stand on the heights.
—Psalm 18:33

Deer can run far without getting tired and climb trails a human can barely see. Each foot has two long toes capped by a hard toenail called a hoof. The outer hoof is hard and gives traction on soft and wet surfaces, while the inner hoof is softer and gives traction on hard surfaces, even cushioning the landing of a jump. Those feet are a miracle of agility and versatility.

God wants to give you mental traction, agility, and resilience so you can climb to the heights. From the heights you will be able to see with new eyes and imagine, "What if my life could be different? What if I could reach the goals I've dreamed of? What if I could leave some old patterns behind and embrace some new ways? What if there could be a big change in the way I care for my physical health? What if my food could come in line and my body could be healed?"

Ask God to give you this new perspective.

FOOD FOR THOUGHT

Whenever you need fresh perspective, ask God to take you up to the heights to see the amazing things that are possible.

REAL LIFE

[Jesus said] "I have come so they may have life. I want them to have it in the
fullest possible way."   —*John 10:10 NIrV*

Jesus wants you to experience the fullness of life. Your relationship with him enables you to pack meaning and purpose into each and every moment. Jesus says this abundant life in him will be better than all your dreams rolled into one.

In this godly life, every part of you is interconnected: your spiritual health is connected to your physical health, and they are both connected to your mental and emotional health. A problem in one area will affect all the others. A new pattern in one area will spread to the other areas.

If you bring all of yourself to God, he will help you change patterns that you may have been stuck in—patterns with food, fitness, or negative thinking, to name a few. Real life in Christ means having the power of his Spirit actively working in you, building full, real life in him.

FOOD FOR THOUGHT

God wants to fill every part of you with real life: physical, mental, emotional, and spiritual wholeness.

DAILY TRUST

"Give us today our daily bread."

—*Matthew 6:11*

Jesus didn't pray, "Give us today our *weekly* bread" or "Give us today our *yearly* bread." You don't need to be concerned about tomorrow until tomorrow. Worrying ahead only distracts us from the steps God has for us to take today.

For instance, you don't need to stress about the future steps necessary to make you Daniel Strong. Focus on what you can do today. Pray for the Holy Spirit to help you do what needs to be done today, and then pray again tomorrow for what you need tomorrow. You can be thankful for what God provides for you today, saying, "Thank you for today's food, today's power, today's new thought pattern."

God wants you to trust him one day at a time. Jesus said, "Give your entire attention to what God is doing right now, and don't get worked up about what may or may not happen tomorrow. God will help you deal with whatever hard things come up when the time comes" (Matthew 6:34 MSG). Isn't that a relief?

FOOD FOR THOUGHT

Trusting God one day at a time frees you from worry and brings true peace.

IT'S UP TO HIM

"The Lord will fight for you; you need only to be still."

—*Exodus 14:14*

The Israelites were fleeing from slavery in Egypt. When they found out that the Egyptian army was pursuing them, they panicked. Moses had to assure them that their survival depended on what God would do, not on their ability to fight for themselves.

God wants you to lay your dreams before him and seek his power to bring them to reality. God "is able to do immeasurably more than all we ask or imagine, according to his power that is at work within us," (Ephesians 3:20). If you can reach your dreams without God, then they're just not big enough. God wants to give you dreams that can only come true through his mighty power.

God will use your dreams to push you beyond your comfort zone. He will use them to keep you from simply settling for so-so results. It may feel risky to dream big, but ultimately your dreams are up to God. He is the one who will fight for them.

FOOD FOR THOUGHT

God will be with you as you step out in faith toward a dream that can only be fulfilled through his mighty power.

RESPONDING TO GOD'S GIFTS

What I'm trying to do here is get you to relax, not be so preoccupied with getting so you can respond to God's giving. People who don't know God and the way he works fuss over these things, but you know both God and how he works.
—Luke 12:29–30 MSG

In the early stages of living the Daniel Plan lifestyle, it's easy to get overwhelmed by the details of what to eat and how to incorporate more movement into our lives. When the process threatens to overwhelm us, it's important to relax and look at the long-range view. It's not all about attaining a certain stage; it's about receiving. As the Bible says, the essential thing is to respond to God's generosity. God has given us an abundance of foods to eat and ways to move. He invites us to enjoy more of his abundance and how he works.

God is so gracious with us. He never pushes us; he invites us to move forward. He leads the way and asks us to follow him. He has infinite patience.

FOOD FOR THOUGHT

Dr. Mark Hyman says, "By adding simple habits—sleeping a bit more, moving your body, calming your mind, breathing, playing, serving—you will gradually, day by day, shift into a profound capacity for self-care and healing."

THE OBEDIENCE THAT COMES FROM FAITH

Blessed are all who fear the LORD, who walk in obedience to him.

—Psalm 128:1

Genuine faith in God always leads to obedience to his commands. The apostle Paul spoke of "the obedience that comes from faith" (Romans 1:5). The apostle John wrote, "And this is love: that we walk in obedience to his commands. As you have heard from the beginning, his command is that you walk in love" (2 John 1:6). To obey God is to love him, and to love him is to obey him.

Your Daniel Plan journey takes you into a life of obedience. The essential of faith moves you to obey God's command to love him with all your heart, soul, mind, and strength. Learning to love foods that love you back and practicing daily movement honor God's command to treat your body as a temple of the Holy Spirit. Focus teaches you to take your thoughts captive to God and shape them according to his thoughts. And friends encourage you to love others as Christ has loved you. The more you follow these practices, the more you will be naturally living in obedience to God's priorities for you.

FOOD FOR THOUGHT

A life of obedience to God's ways is the most free, most liberated life you can imagine.

PERFECT PEACE

You will keep in perfect peace those whose minds are steadfast, because they trust in you.   —*Isaiah 26:3*

As you work to renew your mind, stress will undoubtedly try to pull you away from your goals. The everyday problems often tempt us to make unhealthy choices out of convenience or as a temporary fix for stress.

It can be easy to get stressed out when we focus on our own limited resources instead of focusing on the unlimited resources through our heavenly Father. When we choose to focus on God, he provides perfect peace. We can fix our thoughts on him by meditating on things we know about him or on promises from his Word. For example, he is faithful, he is all-powerful, he is wise. "Your love, LORD, reaches to the heavens, your faithfulness to the skies. Your righteousness is like the highest mountains, your justice like the great deep" (Psalm 36:5–6).

Filling our minds with these truths from his Word will bring peace into our hearts. And peace of mind is the key to beating stress.

FOOD FOR THOUGHT

God's peace is more than enough to lift you above your stress and to reset your mind.

CHASING AWAY FEAR

Well-formed love banishes fear. Since fear is crippling, a fearful life . . .
is one not yet fully formed in love. —1 John 4:18 MSG

Do you avoid getting close to others for fear that if people know what you're really like, you'll be judged or rejected? Or maybe you fear that your fellow Christians expect you to live up to a higher standard of faith and holiness than you can manage.

God's answer to that fear is love. God enables us to love the fear out of one another.

We drive fear from our communities by loving one another so supportively that each person feels safe to open up. This safety allows us to bring our joy and pain, our victories and defeats to others.

Take a step to create community or deepen the one you already have with family, friends, neighbors, or co-workers. For instance, be a safe person for others by supporting them when they suffer setbacks. Take a courageous step of vulnerability by being open about your own ups and downs. Trust that God will use your openness to encourage others. Ask him to drive out your fear and alleviate the fears of others as you offer his love.

FOOD FOR THOUGHT

Let God's love be at the center of your relationships, chasing away fear.

GOD'S STRENGTH SAVES US

This happened that we might not rely on ourselves but on God, who raises the dead.
—2 Corinthians 1:9

God once told Gideon, an Israelite war leader, "You have too many men. I cannot deliver Midian into their hands, or Israel would boast against me, 'My own strength has saved me'" (Judges 7:2). So God whittled Israel's army down from 32,000 to 300 men, so that the odds would be impossible without God's power. God sometimes does a similar thing in our lives to keep us from being able to say, "My own strength has saved me."

God doesn't expect us to be perfect. In fact, he uses our failures to show us that we need him and to drive us into his arms of grace. God sees weakness as a normal part of life. He is not surprised when we stumble on our own. When we fail on our own and succeed only when we utterly depend on him, then he gets the glory. Thus, failure isn't a surprise or a misfortune. It's an opportunity.

FOOD FOR THOUGHT

Failure is a great opportunity to learn to rely more deeply on God, who can turn challenges and obstacles into new life.

CLINGING AND RESTING

"Let the beloved of the LORD rest secure in him, for he shields him all day long, and the one the LORD loves rests between his shoulders."

—Deuteronomy 33:12

Picture a father giving a piggyback ride to a young child. If the child lays down his head, he rests right between dad's shoulders. The fit is just right, intimate and secure. And that's how God longs to carry you. Rest secure in him, because he shields you all day long. Hard times may come, but they are ultimately in the hands of a good and loving God.

We can have such deep intimacy with Christ if we rest securely in him. We can say with the psalmist, "Because you are my help, I sing in the shadow of your wings. I cling to you; your right hand upholds me" (Psalm 63:7–8). He is our rock, our fortress, and our deliverer no matter what is going on in our lives. All we need to do is draw close to him and hold on.

FOOD FOR THOUGHT

Rest securely on God's shoulders, knowing that he shields you all day long.

ESSENTIAL ACCEPTANCE

Accept one another, then, just as Christ accepted you, in order to bring
praise to God. —Romans 15:7

God accepts you with all of your quirks and flaws. When you have a rough day and you make mistakes, he understands that you're in a learning process. He welcomes you no matter how you're feeling at the moment.

That's the kind of acceptance he wants you to have for the people who are supporting you on your journey toward a healthier lifestyle. If you're in a small group or you have a Daniel Plan buddy, you're going to need to accept one another on good days and bad days. You're going to need patience for the other person's less-than-perfect performance, just as he or she will need patience for yours. Acceptance is essential in order for your relationships to be safe enough to help each other grow.

FOOD FOR THOUGHT

Accepting one another in the messiness of life, on good days and bad days, will bring praise to God and will give you a support system you can count on.

OVERCOMING LONELINESS

God places the lonely in families.

—Psalm 68:6 NLT

Everybody feels lonely sometimes. We are all social beings who are designed to need and thrive in community. The community of God's people is a family, and it is meant to be a family that welcomes lonely people and gives them a place where they belong.

If you are facing loneliness, join a group where you have a common interest or call on a friend or family member. It just takes a bit of courage and a decision to be interested in other people.

If loneliness is not at your door right now, consider the lonely people in your world. Reach out to someone who is lonely and offer your companionship. Look for the people who seem to be on the outside, and draw them in. Ask them questions and show a genuine interest in their lives. As you do this, you'll remind the lonely that God is with them—just like he is with you. He is never far. The psalmist said to God, "If I go up to the heavens, you are there; if I make my bed in the depths, you are there" (Psalm 139:8). God always has his eyes on us.

FOOD FOR THOUGHT

God wants to help us have deep, nourishing connections. He will supply our need as we seek him and reach out to others.

BRINGING GOOD OUT OF ANGER

"In your anger do not sin": Do not let the sun go down while you are still angry.
—*Ephesians 4:26*

We all feel anger from time to time. It's a natural response to hurt or threat. We don't have to let anger drive us to make unhealthy choices or act in ways we will later regret. Rather than stuffing it down or lashing out at others, we can constructively address it.

A healthy response to anger begins with saying forthrightly to ourselves, "I'm angry at _____ because _____." We need to admit we're angry. Even if we think the anger is unwarranted or out of proportion, we still need to admit it's there.

Next, we need to identify the hurt or threat behind the anger. Anger can teach us about what we desire, because it often comes from thwarted desire. Desires aren't necessarily sinful, so we don't need to be ashamed to identify the desire that isn't being met. Once we've learned from anger, we ask God how to deal with it.

Are you angry about something? How can you make a fruitful response to your anger?

FOOD FOR THOUGHT

Let anger be a learning opportunity, as well as a chance to understand yourself better and grow more into God's likeness.

TEAMWORK ON A BIG DREAM

Then Solomon began to build the temple of the LORD in Jerusalem on Mount Moriah, where the LORD had appeared to his father David.

—2 Chronicles 3:1

King David had a big dream: to build a temple where the people of Israel could worship God. The Lord allowed David to lay the groundwork for the project, buying the land and stockpiling the materials, but his son Solomon would do the actual building. Solomon had a passion for the project too, and he devoted the early years of his reign to accomplishing it. A huge team of builders and craftsmen worked together to make the magnificent temple a reality.

Has God given you a dream? If your dream is from the Lord, he will work through you to bring it to pass. Most likely you will need a team to help you accomplish it. Don't worry if it's too big a project for you to fulfill on your own; God's power is far beyond yours and a team can do what no individual can.

FOOD FOR THOUGHT

God can turn big dreams into reality, and he often uses a team of people whose hearts are passionately devoted to him.

NO SHAME

Both the one who makes people holy and those who are made holy are of the same family. So Jesus is not ashamed to call them brothers and sisters.

—*Hebrews 2:11*

Jesus is the one who makes people holy, set apart for God's purposes. "Those who are made holy" includes everyone who has put their faith in Christ, including you. If you have surrendered to Christ as your Lord, then he has made you holy, no matter what mistakes you have made. He still delights to call you his brother or sister. You are family.

Jesus doesn't want shame to interfere with your growth. Shame can cause you to doubt your identity as a child of the Father. Doubt leads to a downward spiral and can derail your efforts to grow and become all God intends for you. So the Bible emphasizes that Jesus will never ever be ashamed of you; he boasts that you are part of his family. "I will be a Father to you, and you will be my sons and daughters, says the Lord Almighty" (2 Corinthians 6:18). That's the core of who you are.

FOOD FOR THOUGHT

Jesus is proud to call you his brother or his sister.

CHOCK-FULL

*The ravens brought him bread and meat in the morning and bread and meat
in the evening, and he drank from the brook.* —*1 Kings 17:6*

In the time of the prophet Elijah, God sent a drought to Israel to
punish the nation for worshiping false gods. There was famine in
the land, but God took care of Elijah. For a while, God actually sent
ravens to Elijah with food twice a day. Then, when the brook where
he was camped dried up, Elijah traveled outside Israel and lived with
a penniless widow. While he was there, her supplies of oil and flour
were miraculously extended so that they never ran out. Elijah didn't
eat like a king, but he and the widow and her son had enough food to
keep them alive for three years.

Most of us don't face going hungry or even a limited food supply,
but God is still Lord of our food, and he cares about our nourishment.
"All creatures look to you to give them their food at the proper time"
(Psalm 104:27). Just as Elijah was thankful for the ravens that fed
him, so we can thank God for the many ways he provides for us.

FOOD FOR THOUGHT

Out of his abundance, God will provide nourishment
so we have the energy to live for and serve him.

FINDING COMFORT

Blessed are those who mourn, for they will be comforted.

—Matthew 5:4

Grief is letting go of something we've lost. It's saying, "Goodbye. I can't keep you. You've left me." If our health has left us, we say goodbye to it. If we've lost a business, we say goodbye to the financial security. If a person has died, we say goodbye to that relationship. This saying goodbye is necessary for our well-being. The function of grief is that it gives us an outlet for our sadness and loss. Without it, we can actually get stuck in anxiety, depression, or anger. Grief says, "I've got to empty out the pain so that I can eventually move on."

Weeping and other physical expressions of grief actually help us renew our minds. Weeping helps us let go and move on. If you have suffered a loss that you haven't gotten over, consider doing something physical to honor that loss. Consider talking to a friend about it. We are able to move through grief when we share it with another person.

FOOD FOR THOUGHT

Mourning is a part of life. Comfort comes when we pour out our grief through tears and allow a friend to meet us in the midst of it.

MULTIPLIED MEALS

They all ate and were satisfied, and the disciples picked up twelve basketfuls of broken pieces that were left over. The number of those who ate was about five thousand men, besides women and children.

—Matthew 14:20–21

A crowd of people followed Jesus to a deserted place to hear him teach. Toward the end of the day, there they all were, far from any place to buy dinner. So Jesus multiplied five barley loaves and two fish into a meal to feed thousands.

Although this seems like an incredible miracle, in fact, God multiplies food for us every day. He is the one who enables a few seeds to become an orchard of apples or a field of ripe tomatoes. At his command, one chicken lays eggs that become many chickens. God does these wonders over time, but the power and the generosity are the same as what Jesus did. This is why we thank God for every meal, because he is ultimately the one putting food on our tables.

Thank God when you buy food, when you prepare it, and when you eat it. A heart of gratitude can revolutionize your attitude to food, especially real food that grows on plants that God made.

FOOD FOR THOUGHT

The reason to eat real food is not to fit in your jeans, but to be awake to the beauty and miracle of life and God's abundant provision.

BUILDING ON ROCK

[Jesus said,] "Everyone who hears my words and puts them into practice is like a wise man. He builds his house on the rock."

—Matthew 7:24 NIrV

Jesus told a parable that asks a question: What are you building your life on? The parable illustrates the wisdom of obedience and the foolishness of disregarding Jesus' words.

As we seek to create a healthier lifestyle, we want to build that lifestyle on the bedrock of Jesus' teaching, honoring how he made our bodies, minds, and relationships to work. Loving God and our neighbor lies at the core of that teaching. If we put God first in everything we do and invest love in the people around us, we will rest on a solid foundation. The storms of life will inevitably come, but they won't flatten what we've built.

So what's the foundation of your life and your health? How are you honoring the way God made you? How can you make love more of a priority?

FOOD FOR THOUGHT

When the rains and wind of life beat against your house, you will weather the storm with God and his love at the center of your life.

REFRESHING OTHERS

Anyone who gives a lot will succeed. Anyone who renews others will be renewed.
—*Proverbs 11:25 NIrV*

We have received so much from God: insights on how to live a healthier life, power from his Holy Spirit to do what we couldn't do in ourselves, support from friends, provision for our needs, grace for our sins. Deliberately counting our blessings is energizing and motivates us to give back to God and our communities.

What is God calling you to do to give back? How can you build up the body of Christ or reach out to people who don't yet know Christ? The more we give, the more we receive so we can give still more. This is true with emotional and relational support, too. The apostle Paul said that God "comforts us in all our troubles so that we can comfort those in any trouble" (2 Corinthians 1:4). The cycle of blessing builds as we give generously and receive gratefully.

FOOD FOR THOUGHT

"If we pray, we will believe; if we believe, we will love; if we love, we will serve." —Unknown

WEALTH IN ACTION

Command them to do good, to be rich in good deeds, and to be generous and willing to share. —1 Timothy 6:18

We have put our "hope in God, who richly provides us with everything for our enjoyment" (1 Timothy 6:17). We're in the process of experiencing the abundance of food, learning to take joy in movement, reaching out to build supportive friends, and growing in our ability to focus on true and beneficial thoughts. More and more, as we move forward on our journey, we must look for ways to give to others what we've learned and experienced.

We're not saved by doing good deeds, but we are saved and transformed so we will be able to do good in the world. There are so many opportunities to love others as we have been loved. Do you know anyone who would benefit from hearing about the Five Essentials of The Daniel Plan? Is there some area of service you want to take on now that you have more health and energy? "Freely you have received; freely give" (Matthew 10:8). Did you ever guess that you'd have so much to give away?

FOOD FOR THOUGHT

It's exhilarating to be generous with the abundance we have received from God.

DANCING HAPPY

Then Miriam the prophet, Aaron's sister, took a timbrel in her hand, and all the women followed her, with timbrels and dancing. Miriam sang to them: "Sing to the LORD, for he is highly exalted. Both horse and driver he has hurled into the sea." —*Exodus 15:20–21*

Dancing was common in Israelite life. People lifted their hearts in worship and celebrated with their bodies by dancing. Miriam led the women in dancing after the Israelites escaped Egypt. God had parted the Red Sea so they could cross it on foot, and when they realized they were safe, they danced.

King David danced when the Ark of the Covenant was transported to Jerusalem. "Wearing a linen ephod, David was dancing before the LORD with all his might, while he and all Israel were bringing up the ark of the LORD with shouts and the sound of trumpets" (2 Samuel 6:14–15).

Dancing is one of the many forms of movement we can use to express joy. What movement do you enjoy? What expresses celebration for you? Consider making celebratory movement more a part of your life.

FOOD FOR THOUGHT

Strengthen your own joy and celebrate God's mighty acts.

DOING GOOD

For we are God's handiwork, created in Christ Jesus to do good works, which God prepared in advance for us to do. —*Ephesians 2:10*

The Bible tells us we are saved by grace, not by works (Ephesians 2:8–9). But we are created to *do* good works. It was never God's intention for us to accept his grace and then sit around. God has planned good acts for us to do long before we are even aware of them. So even though we're not saved by good works, we are saved *for* them. It is our privilege to partner with the Holy Spirit in doing good in the world. In truth, it is our destiny.

Part of the joy of getting healthy is that we'll find ourselves far more able and energized to do all we were created for. What are those things God created for you to do? What are the unique contributions to God's kingdom that you can make this week, this month, this year?

FOOD FOR THOUGHT

You are God's handiwork—his unique work of art—that he has created to do good in the world.

SLEEP ENERGY

In peace I will lie down and sleep, for you alone, LORD, make me dwell in safety.
                                        —Psalm 4:8

Sleep is God's gift. To accept that gift is an act of trust. He restores your body and energy through sleep.

One of the hidden triggers to overeating is lack of rest. When we are overtired, we often try to boost our energy with caffeine, sugar, or carbs. That ultimately makes us more tired than before.

Jesus understood the value of rest. When his disciples returned to him after a long ministry trip, they found him in the thick of ministry himself. "Because so many people were coming and going that they did not even have a chance to eat, [Jesus] said to them, 'Come with me by yourselves to a quiet place and get some rest'" (Mark 6:31). Jesus needed rest, and his disciples needed it even more. Rest ultimately gives us more energy to accomplish all the priorities God has for each of us.

FOOD FOR THOUGHT

God makes us lie down in green pastures (Psalm 23:2) so that we can rise up again refreshed and restored.

THE CHRIST MINDSET

Have the same mind-set as Christ Jesus.

—*Philippians 2:5*

Changing your health habits is like driving a speedboat on a lake with your autopilot set to go east when you want to head west. If you want to reverse course, you could try to physically force the wheel in the opposite direction, but you would likely get tired and let go, and the boat would drift back east.

There is a better option: Change your autopilot. Your mind is your autopilot, and the best way to change your habits for the long term is to change the way you think. You need a new mindset, the mind-set of Christ.

Through his Holy Spirit and his Word, God gives us "divine power to demolish strongholds" (2 Corinthians 10:4). Strongholds are deeply rooted ways of thinking, and they can be demolished when we meditate on God's Word and ask him to replace lies with his truth. We can ask, "Father, what would Jesus think about this matter?" Or "Lord, please show me the false things I believe that are getting in the way of my health and growth."

FOOD FOR THOUGHT

If we immerse ourselves in God's Word, the mindset of Christ will free us to change our autopilot and change our lives.

EXERCISING YOUR EARS

To answer before listening—that is folly and shame.

—*Proverbs 18:13*

To be a good friend, we need to learn to be good listeners. We need to let people tell us a whole story or express their thoughts and emotions before we jump in with advice. Often, advice isn't what people need. They may know what they need to do; they just need the strength that comes from being truly heard and understood. They may need to tell someone their fears before they can overcome them with faith.

Consider this: God patiently listens to you, even though he already knows what you are going to say. He doesn't cut you off or rush you through your thoughts. He's not afraid of your anger, and his response is thoughtful and in your best interest. If the God of the universe does this for you, should you do any less for your friends?

James tells us to be quick to listen and slow to speak (James 1:19). The most loving thing we can do for someone is often to provide a listening ear.

FOOD FOR THOUGHT

"Friendship is one of the sweetest joys of life. Many might have failed beneath the bitterness of their trial had they not found a friend."—Charles Spurgeon[23]

THE MODEL OF JESUS

*I reach out for your commands that I love. I do this so that I may think
deeply about your orders.* —*Psalm 119:48 NIrV*

The temptation to abandon the healthy habits you are learning can be strong at times. The most reliable way to resist that temptation is to follow the model of Jesus. Matthew 4:1–11 tells us that when Jesus was tempted, he responded with Scripture.

Jesus memorized and thought about Scripture. Thinking about a verse and repeating it to ourselves until we remember it is such a gift of life. For example, we might meditate on Colossians 1:10–11, "We pray that you will grow to know God better. We want you to be very strong, in keeping with his glorious power" (NIrV). Just praying that verse opens the door for the Holy Spirit to reframe our thoughts and fill us with that strength. Or if we're facing a setback, we can meditate on 2 Corinthians 4:16: "We do not lose heart. Though outwardly we are wasting away, yet inwardly we are being renewed day by day."

FOOD FOR THOUGHT

No habit will help you more in the spiritual dynamics of getting healthy than memorizing and meditating on the Word of God.

GENEROUS MEASURES

Give, and it will be given to you. A good measure, pressed down, shaken together and running over, will be poured into your lap.

—Luke 6:38

When we find a way to serve others even while we are in the process of getting healthy, we add to our joy. Helping other people actually stimulates the brain chemicals that make us feel happiness.

When our focus is completely on ourselves, it's easy for our lives to get stagnant. But when we're giving, we become like a lake where fresh water flows in one end and out the other, nourishing both the life in the lake and the life downstream.

Generosity to others widens our hearts and makes it easier for God to be generous with us. Where is there a need around you? If you ask God to show you an area where you can give back out of gratitude for what you've received, he'll be delighted to respond.

FOOD FOR THOUGHT

God will pour into us abundantly when we give abundantly to others.

SPECIALIZED GIFTS

Everything you are and think and do is permeated with Oneness. But that doesn't mean you should all look and speak and act the same. Out of the generosity of Christ, each of us is given his own gift.

—Ephesians 4:6–7 MSG

We are all parts of one body, the body of Christ, yet each of us is unique. We each have a unique contribution to make to the work of God in the world. And we are happiest when we are using the abilities God gave us to accomplish something worthwhile. We're designed to be others-centered, not self-centered. We long to live meaningful lives.

The Bible says, "Each of you should use whatever gift you have received to serve others, as faithful stewards of God's grace in its various forms" (1 Peter 4:10). What are your strengths? What opportunities do you have to help others? You don't have to reach your health goals before you start giving back; in fact, giving back will energize you to take better care of yourself, just as taking better care of yourself will energize you to give.

FOOD FOR THOUGHT

Out of God's incredible generosity, he has given unique strengths to you to encourage and influence others.

OUR DOUBTS

Jesus said, "Everything is possible for one who believes." Immediately the boy's father exclaimed, "I do believe; help me overcome my unbelief!"
—Mark 9:23–24

Confronting destructive lifelong habits and working toward better physical health can be one of the scariest things some people experience in their lives. Faith is believing that God can do the seemingly impossible in your life, even if you don't understand how.

When this father asked Jesus to heal his son, he believed in Jesus but was honest enough to say, "Help me with my doubts!" Believing in Jesus doesn't mean we never have any doubts or fears. We can keep taking our doubts and fears to him over and over, and he will continue to embrace us and change us, doubts and all.

"Now faith is confidence in what we hope for and assurance about what we do not see" (Hebrews 11:1). God will reward the faith and understand the doubts, and gradually our courage and trust in him will grow.

FOOD FOR THOUGHT

God longs to help us with our doubts so that we can step forward without fear.

FOOD FESTIVAL

For seven days celebrate the festival to the LORD your God at the place
the LORD will choose. For the LORD your God will bless you in all your
harvest and in all the work of your hands, and your joy will be complete.
—Deuteronomy 16:15

Ancient Israel's calendar had several major festivals that celebrated events in Israel's history as well as annual events in the agricultural year. For example, the Festival of Tabernacles commemorated the earlier time when the people lived in huts in the wilderness, and it also celebrated the end of the fruit harvest each year. Tabernacles was a seven-day feast with special foods. It gave the people a chance to thank God for the harvest of the current year and to pray for rain for the coming year. Managers and workers alike shared in the feast, and joy was the reigning attitude.

We no longer officially celebrate harvest times, and we can feel distant from the sources of our food. But if we eat real food that God made, we can thank him for the harvest, for the workers who grow the food, and for the water that makes the plants grow. Each meal can be a festival celebrating God's goodness.

FOOD FOR THOUGHT

Eating is a sacred experience that can connect us to our senses, our bodies, one another, and the God who provides the food we share.

BROADEN YOUR HORIZON

None of you should look out just for your own good. Each of you should
also look out for the good of others. —Philippians 2:4 NIrV

It's natural to focus on yourself when you're trying to make lifestyle changes. Yet part of growing to be like Jesus is taking the focus off yourself and caring about others. The Bible says to look to others' interests and not just your own.

Focusing on yourself and your health journey eventually narrows your perspective. This can lead you to believe your challenges are worse than anyone else's, which can lead to discouragement.

But when you broaden your horizon and pay attention to others' needs, you find that everybody is struggling with something. You see the progress others are making, and that gives you hope for your own progress. You realize you're not alone, and neither are your friends. When they face a fork in the road and need discernment, offering them help is a great way to put their needs ahead of yours. And when you selflessly work for their success, you gain encouragement from their triumphs just as if they were your own.

FOOD FOR THOUGHT

If you help others get ahead, you find yourself celebrating victories beyond what you could expect for yourself alone.

BREATH AND LIFE

He himself gives everyone life and breath and everything else.... God did this so that they would seek him and perhaps reach out for him and find him, though he is not far from any one of us. "For in him we live and move and have our being." —Acts 17:25, 27–28

Breath comes from God. Whenever we move, we are moving his creation. There is a special holiness to breath and movement. If we breathe slowly, we become more conscious of his presence filling us. And if we move mindfully, we can celebrate the way our bodies move in so many ways. Connect faith with fitness. For example, when we walk, we can think about what it means to walk with God. When we stretch, we can use that as a cue to reflect on what we're thankful for.

The psalmist prays, "We will never turn our back on you; breathe life into our lungs so we can shout your name!" (Psalm 80:18 MSG).

FOOD FOR THOUGHT

It's awe-inspiring to know that God is as near to us as our breath, upholding us in every movement.

NEVER FINAL

The Lord makes secure the footsteps of the person who delights in him, even if that person trips, he won't fall. The Lord's hand takes good care of him.
—Psalm 37:23–24 NIrV

Picture the Lord directing your steps and delighting in every detail of your life. Even if you stumble, you will stand up again, because the Lord is holding your hand.

Under this scenario, failure is never final. You haven't failed if you don't reach one of your goals, because there is no end date. You have simply stumbled, and you can get up again. If you overdo it on a dessert or miss an opportunity to move your body, tomorrow is a new day. Mistakes are simply lessons in what doesn't work so you can get closer to what does work. Mistakes are chances to build your faith by experiencing again that you are weak but God is strong enough to lift you up.

As you grow in wisdom, you'll discover that "When you walk, your steps will not be hampered; when you run, you will not stumble" (Proverbs 4:12). Gradually, you'll stumble less and less until you are running on the pathway God has laid out for you.

FOOD FOR THOUGHT

The Lord holds your hand, delighting in every detail of your journey.

JESUS UNDERSTANDS

*We don't have a priest who is out of touch with our reality. He's been
through weakness and testing, experienced it all—all but the sin. So let's
walk right up to him and get what he is so ready to give. Take the mercy,
accept the help.* —Hebrews 4:15–16 MSG

Jesus understands the temptation to get discouraged and give up on
our goals. During his earthly life, he experienced that same temptation. He never quit, but he experienced the temptation to quit. That's
why he doesn't get impatient with us. He knows what it's like, and he's
more than ready to help us to resist temptation and give his mercy
when we do give in, quit, and need to begin again. We never run out of
chances for a fresh start.

Jesus voluntarily took on weakness and humanity for our sakes.
That's how much he loves us. He wanted us never to doubt that he
knows what we're going through. Sometimes it may feel like God is
far removed from our struggles, like he doesn't care, but that's not
true. He's in the struggle with us, carrying us through and strengthening us.

FOOD FOR THOUGHT

Christ's love is extravagant; he doesn't love in order
to get something from us but to give everything of
himself to us (Ephesians 5:2).

FORGIVING OURSELVES

If you, Lord, kept a record of sins, Lord, who could stand? But with you there is forgiveness, so that we can, with reverence, serve you.

—Psalm 130:3–4

God doesn't keep a record of your sins. Instead, he forgives them, because Jesus carried all of them on the cross. And if he doesn't keep an account of your sins, he certainly expects you to put them behind you, too. Yesterday's mistakes are over; today is a fresh start.

Sometimes, even though we know about God's forgiveness, we have trouble forgiving ourselves when we hit a snag. We may rehearse our mistakes and pile on the blame. That's not the way God deals with us. There is no condemnation in him. So we can say to ourselves, "God keeps no record of my mistakes, and I can let go of them, too."

Do you tend to pile on the self-criticism? Ask God to help you let go of that habit and believe forgiveness is for every sin, every time.

FOOD FOR THOUGHT

God keeps no record of our sins and mistakes; we are completely and thoroughly forgiven.

FORGIVING OTHERS

If you forgive other people when they sin against you, your heavenly Father will also forgive you.　　　　　　　　　　　　　*—Matthew 6:14*

Life is messy. Other people fall short just as we do. As often as we need to receive forgiveness, we also need to give it. The prayer that Jesus modeled for us says, "Forgive us our debts, as we also have forgiven our debtors" (Matthew 6:12). Over and over he says that the measure we use for others will be used on us: "Do not condemn, and you will not be condemned. Forgive, and you will be forgiven" (Luke 6:37).

"Peter came to Jesus and asked, 'Lord, how many times shall I forgive my brother or sister who sins against me? Up to seven times?' Jesus answered, 'I tell you, not seven times, but seventy-seven times'" (Matthew 18:21–22).

When it's hard to forgive, we can reflect on the many times Jesus has forgiven us. What a joy it is that we don't have to carry that burden. Pass along the joy of releasing other people from similar burdens. Forgiveness lifts a huge weight from our shoulders.

FOOD FOR THOUGHT

We have received abundant mercy, so let's be merciful, just as our Father is merciful (Luke 6:36).

SHAPED FOR A PURPOSE

From his dwelling place he watches all who live on earth—he who forms the hearts of all, who considers everything they do. —Psalm 33:14–15

God is paying attention to what you do with your life. He's looking to see what you do with what he's given you. But he's not going to do everything for you.

Think about Joseph. Could Joseph the herdsman have guessed that he would one day be the number two man in Egypt's government, protecting a whole nation from famine (Genesis 37–47)? Joseph got to that position by being a good steward of the gifts God had given him, gifts of managing his masters' affairs and even the gift of interpreting dreams. When he helped a fellow prisoner one day, it became a turning point in his life.

This journey toward health isn't an end in itself. You're getting healthy so that you have the vitality to do all God has designed you to do. God has a unique journey planned for you, and you just need to step out in faith and begin.

FOOD FOR THOUGHT

God joyfully watches everything you do, eager to see you use the gifts he has given you.

SERVE ONE ANOTHER

Each of you should use whatever gift you have received to serve others, as faithful stewards of God's grace in its various forms. —*1 Peter 4:10*

One of the best ways you can express your gratitude for what you've learned from the Daniel Plan is to find ways to use your gifts to build up other people. If you've learned to cook, help someone else learn the basics. Help someone clean out their pantry, invite someone to join you for a workout class, host a dinner party with Daniel Plan foods, or write encouraging notes to the members of your small group. When the receiving leads to more giving, you are responding to God in the way he desires.

Even more important, spread the good news about Jesus and build up God's family. Jesus says, "But seek first his kingdom and his righteousness, and all these things will be given to you as well" (Matthew 6:33). The highest priority you can give your life to is the kingdom of God. When you serve, you give gratitude to God for the many blessings you have received from him through others.

FOOD FOR THOUGHT

Your life will be incalculably richer if you're giving away what you've received.

A TOUGH ONE

"Today I have made you a fortified city, an iron pillar and a bronze wall to stand against the whole land—against the kings of Judah, its officials, its priests and the people of the land. They will fight against you but will not overcome you, for I am with you and will rescue you," declares the LORD.
—Jeremiah 1:18–19

God gave Jeremiah a tough assignment: he had to prophesy about the disaster coming upon the nation. He had to repeatedly proclaim what the leaders and people of his country didn't want to hear. So God gave him a thick skin; he was tough, "a fortified city, an iron pillar and a bronze wall." He had what it took to be diligent and persistent.

We need diligence and persistence like Jeremiah's if we're going to reach our health goals and the dreams God is calling us to. Like Jeremiah, we need to keep getting up when we're knocked down. We need to press through resistance. We need to keep going day after day. God wants to give us that diligence and persistence, and he'll hear us when we pray for it.

FOOD FOR THOUGHT

God will give you the diligence and persistence to pursue the life he is designing for you.

SHARE THE LOAD

"Come to me, all you who are weary and burdened, and I will give you rest. Take my yoke upon you and learn from me, for I am gentle and humble in heart, and you will find rest for your souls. For my yoke is easy and my burden is light." —Matthew 11:28–30

A yoke is a wooden bar or frame that is put over the necks of two oxen so they can pull one cart together. When Jesus says, "Take my yoke upon you," he's saying, "Stop trying to pull that cart by yourself. It's too heavy for you. Instead, you and I will be yoked together, and I'll help you pull that load. I know where we're going and how fast we should go. And I have the strength you don't have on your own."

If your health goals have you feeling weary and burdened, maybe it's because you're trying to accomplish them on your own. Let Jesus come alongside you and share the load. Ask him. He'll be glad to be yoked to you on this journey.

FOOD FOR THOUGHT

When we're yoked together with Jesus, our burden is light, and he provides rest for our weary souls.

FACING DELAYS

You have joy even though you may have had to suffer for a little while. You may have had to suffer sadness in all kinds of trouble. Your troubles have come in order to prove that your faith is real. Your faith is worth more than gold. That's because gold can pass away even when fire has made it pure.

—1 Peter 1:6–7 NIrV

Abraham had to wait decades for God to fulfill his promise of a son. God often makes us wait for the things he has promised so that our faith builds in the waiting. The prophet Habakkuk got a vision from God about the future, and he had to wait for its fulfillment. God said, "It might take a while. But wait for it. You can be sure it will come. It will happen when I want it to" (Habakkuk 2:3 NIrV).

If you have a picture of where you want to be when you reach your health goals, don't give up in the face of difficulties and delays. These occur to prove your faith, to teach you to rely on God, and to motivate you to trust God's timetable. Proven faith is far more precious than gold.

Are you waiting for God to act? If you're doing everything you need to do, then you can relax and wait with confidence.

FOOD FOR THOUGHT

Wait patiently for God's answer; your victory comes from him (Psalm 62:1).

MOVED TO GRATITUDE

Even though I was once a blasphemer and a persecutor and a violent man,
I was shown mercy because I acted in ignorance and unbelief.

—1 Timothy 1:13

Before he came to faith in Christ, the apostle Paul was one of the chief persecutors of Jesus' followers. He dragged many to prison and participated in the murder of Stephen. Yet once Paul came to believe in Christ, he didn't let his past weigh him down. He accepted the forgiveness God offered. He wrote, "Christ Jesus came into the world to save sinners—of whom I am the worst. But for that very reason I was shown mercy so that in me, the worst of sinners, Christ Jesus might display his immense patience as an example for those who would believe in him and receive eternal life" (1 Timothy 1:15–16).

Sometimes we have difficulty letting go of our mistakes. We criticize ourselves for them, and we let them keep us from living joyfully in the present. We may think that because we haven't been able to overcome our challenges in the past, there is no hope for us. But Paul simply let his past move him to gratitude for God's mercy. Let's do the same.

FOOD FOR THOUGHT

Our past missteps can motivate us to deeper gratitude for God's generous redemption.

SABBATH REST

Six days you shall labor, but on the seventh day you shall rest; even during the plowing season and harvest you must rest. —*Exodus 34:21*

Rest is so important to God that he made ten percent of the Ten Commandments about it. The Sabbath is one day out of seven when the people of God are told to rest from their work and to let everybody who works for them rest too.

When the Israelites first received the Ten Commandments, they were trekking across the desert, and God trained them to rest. God sent no manna on the Sabbath, so they had nothing to do but rest. But when they got to the Promised Land and began farming, they quickly began to struggle with the idea of leaving their labor for a Sabbath every week, especially during seasons like the harvest, when every hour counted.

We're similar. During our busy seasons, we can have trouble trusting God with our work. We may take a day off from the office, but then we take work home or do the chores that have been piling up.

God asks us to trust him enough to take time off. He knows we'll be at our best during the other six days if we get a break.

FOOD FOR THOUGHT

If you plan rest into your week to rejuvenate your body and spirit, your life will be far richer and more energized.

I SHAPED YOU

I have made you, you are my servant; Israel, I will not forget you.
—Isaiah 44:21

God is for you. He's not against you, and he's not indifferent. He made you and shaped you just the way he wanted you to be. None of your strengths and weaknesses, nothing about your body, none of it is a mistake. He says you are one who is "called by my name, whom I created for my glory, whom I formed and made" (Isaiah 43:7).

If you're naturally quiet and thrive with just a few close friends, that's God's design for you. If you find joy in walking and your body can't handle running, that's the way God shaped you. Embrace the way you're made.

Whatever challenges you are facing as you seek to reach your health goals, he says, "Do not fear, for I have redeemed you; I have summoned you by name; you are mine" (Isaiah 43:1). Consider meditating on these truths so that they sink deep into your soul.

FOOD FOR THOUGHT

God formed you, made you, shaped you just the way he wants you to be, and you have the privilege of living out that shape as you continue to walk in him.

TRUE THOUGHTS

Whatever is true, whatever is noble, whatever is right, whatever is pure, whatever is lovely, whatever is admirable—if anything is excellent or praiseworthy—think about such things. —Philippians 4:8

What do you fill your mind with? The Bible says to fill it with what is true, with what is noble, with excellent and praiseworthy things. Why? Because you become what you think about. Pastor Rick Warren says that whatever gets your attention gets you. Proverbs tells us to be careful how we think because our thoughts shape our life (Proverbs 4:23).

If you fill your mind with true thoughts, you become more grounded in reality. If you fill it with noble thoughts, you become nobler. You become purer, lovelier, more admirable and excellent and praiseworthy in your actions because you tend to act on what you think about long enough.

The Bible is a good source of true and noble thoughts. Meditating on its truths will make your mind and your life richer.

FOOD FOR THOUGHT

Because you tend to do and become what you think about, refresh yourself by setting your mind on true, noble, and admirable thoughts.

YOUR CREATIVE BEST

*Make a careful exploration of who you are and the work you have
been given, and then sink yourself into that . . . Each of you must take
responsibility for doing the creative best you can with your own life.*
　　　　　　　　　　　　　　　—Galatians 6:4–5 MSG

D oing your creative best means to develop all that God created
you to be. The goal is not to change who you are; it's to work
with exactly who you are.

How has God shaped you? What work has he given you? Those
are the kinds of questions the apostle Paul urges you to ask yourself.
The Bible says God formed you the way a potter forms clay into a
variety of utensils, each with different uses. "Yet you, LORD, are our
Father. We are the clay, you are the potter; we are all the work of your
hand" (Isaiah 64:8). Pay attention to the abilities and skills he has
blessed you with so you can do the creative best with your life.

FOOD FOR THOUGHT

Who you are and the work you have been given in
the world matter deeply to God, who has a good plan
for your life as you leave your imprint on the world
around you.

WORRY PRAYERS

Don't fret or worry. Instead of worrying, pray. Let petitions and praises shape your worries into prayers, letting God know your concerns.
—Philippians 4:6 MSG

Worrying changes nothing, but prayer and worship connect you with the all-powerful God who loves to hear and respond. Reframing a worry into a prayer will transform the way you think about your situation, and thinking differently will lower your stress.

What can you praise God for in the midst of a circumstance that tempts you to worry? Worship will raise your heart above the circumstance and help you see God. The psalmist cries out, "Let all who take refuge in you be glad; let them ever sing for joy. Spread your protection over them, that those who love your name may rejoice in you" (Psalm 5:11).

He will help you. He promises to be right there with you whenever you call on him. The Bible says, "If you don't know what you're doing, pray to the Father. He loves to help" (James 1:5 MSG).

FOOD FOR THOUGHT

Praying is often the most fruitful thing you can do, because it brings the all-powerful God into a situation and changes your mindset.

TWO-WAY TRUST

The One I've trusted in can take care of what he's trusted me to do right
to the end. —2 Timothy 1:12 MSG

God has trusted you to do certain things in the world. Yet he hasn't just given you these tasks and walked away. The apostle Paul said God is actively involved. You can trust him to help you do what he's entrusted to you.

Even if you feel as though a task is beyond your ability to accomplish, reach out to God, knowing that he will take care of it. He's designed it to be beyond what you can do on your own so that you'll trust in him.

God values your trust more than anything else you could give him. He wants you—all of you, spiritual and physical—surrendered to him. That's why he's invited you on this journey toward health. He wants you healthy, but even more, he wants your heart surrendered to him in utter dependence.

FOOD FOR THOUGHT

Whatever tasks are before you, find new hope by entrusting them completely to the One who has entrusted them to you.

YOU'RE CALLED

We never stop praying for you. Our God has chosen you. We pray that he will make you worthy of his choice. We pray he will make every good thing you want to do come true. We pray that he will do this by his power.
— 2 Thessalonians 1:11 NIrV

Your faith is prompting you to do all sorts of good things. That's what real faith does. Some of those good things may seem beyond your reach, but don't give up! Pray instead that God will give you the power to accomplish them. He is "able to do immeasurably more than all we ask or imagine, according to his power that is at work within us" (Ephesians 3:20).

What might happen if you and your friends consistently prayed for each other to live worthy of God's call? What might you accomplish? Pause to let yourself dream. Don't worry about being too grandiose. Just picture what a life worthy of God's call might look like. You can't make it happen in your own strength, so there's no pressure on you. God will empower you to do it. Let him plant the vision inside you.

FOOD FOR THOUGHT

A life worthy of God's call—through his strength—is the richest way to live.

ORDINARY AND EXTRAORDINARY

We have this treasure in jars of clay to show that this all-surpassing power is from God and not from us. —2 Corinthians 4:7

You're like a clay pot filled with diamonds. Ordinary but containing something extraordinary: the message about who Jesus is and what he has done. You are part of God's "chosen people, [his] royal priesthood, [his] holy nation, God's special possession, that you may declare the praises of him who called you out of darkness into his wonderful light" (1 Peter 2:9). God made your body and your mind for this purpose: that you might declare his praises.

And he made you ordinary so that when he does extraordinary things through you, all the credit and glory go to him. God is the one with incomparable power, and he wants to exercise it through you.

That's the reason he wants to help you get healthy. He has a plan for your life, and you need all your vitality to accomplish it.

FOOD FOR THOUGHT

You may be ordinary, but you carry with you something extraordinary, the good news about what Christ has done for you and the rest of the world.

GOD'S INVITATION

So because of God's mercy, we have work to do. He has given it to us. And
we don't give up. —2 *Corinthians 4:1 NIrV*

God has generously let us in on what he's doing in the world. He's put his Holy Spirit in us and invited us to join him in spreading his kingdom throughout the world. He's invited us to get healthy enough to participate in this magnificent venture.

So we're not about to quit and walk off the job just because the process of getting healthy is occasionally difficult. The apostle Paul endured a "thorn in [his] flesh" (2 Corinthians 12:7) throughout his ministry, and he embraced it because it was his calling. He was confident that it was the most satisfying life he could possibly live. We, too, can persevere in our callings because God is behind them and strengthens us day by day. Sharing in God's kingdom work is the highest honor we could have.

FOOD FOR THOUGHT

God is strengthening us so that we can participate in the glorious work he's doing, spreading the amazing news of his kingdom throughout the world.

WILLING?

When we see that you're just as willing to endure the hard times as to enjoy the good times, we know you're going to make it, no doubt about it.

—*2 Corinthians 1:7 MSG*

There are days when the process of changing lifelong habits feels incredibly difficult. Billy Graham said, "Each life is made up of mistakes and learning, waiting and growing, practicing patience and being persistent."[24]

God will provide the strength to endure; all he asks us to provide is the willingness. When hard moments hit, we can refresh our hearts with deep draughts of God's Word. The Bible says, "God has breathed life into all Scripture. It is useful for teaching us what is true. It is useful for correcting our mistakes. It is useful for making our lives whole again" (2 Timothy 3:16 NIrV). It's one of the most important tools God uses to carry us through change and growth.

We can also take time to be alone with God, drinking in his goodness, and time with friends, letting their encouragement be God's voice to us. What is your favorite way to tap into God for endurance?

FOOD FOR THOUGHT

You're going to make it through the hard moments of the change process, because God is right there with you, giving you the endurance you need.

WHO'S DRIVING?

Anyone who intends to come with me has to let me lead. You're not in the driver's seat; I am. Don't run from suffering; embrace it. Follow me and I'll show you how. —Matthew 16:24 MSG

Jesus asked his disciples to hand over the keys of their lives to him. After they saw him raised from the dead, they were willing to follow him anywhere, even into suffering.

Sometimes we still struggle with wanting to be in the driver's seat, but we won't get anywhere that way. When we hand over the keys to Jesus, we'll run away from the hard parts of the change process less and less. Instead, we'll embrace them. "We are transfigured much like the Messiah, our lives gradually becoming brighter and more beautiful as God enters our lives and we become like him" (2 Corinthians 3:18 MSG).

What hard situation is Jesus asking you to embrace this week? You don't have to endure it in your own strength. Let him drive.

FOOD FOR THOUGHT

Let Jesus take the driver's seat in your life. As you follow him, your life will shine more and more with his holy character.

MUTUAL ENCOURAGEMENT

I want us to encourage one another in the faith we share.

—Romans 1:12 NirV

E ven the apostle Paul needed encouragement from his fellow believers. He understood that God didn't design us to be alone or apart from the body of Christ. In fact, the Bible says, "It is not good for the man to be alone" (Genesis 2:18). God created us as relational beings. We need support from a colleague or a small group, a spouse or a friend.

People give us essential nutrients that we need to grow, nutrients like support, validation, comfort, enthusiasm, empathy, sympathy, wisdom, and feedback. It's far easier to grow if we get these nutrients that are found only in relationships.

Who in your life offers you those nutrients? Who do you know who needs those nutrients from you? Relationships are designed to be mutual, so if you start giving encouragement away, it is likely to come back to you as well.

FOOD FOR THOUGHT

The nutrients that come only through relationships will help you lead a well-nourished, rich, and satisfying life.

FIX YOUR THOUGHTS ON JESUS

Therefore, holy brothers and sisters, who share in the heavenly calling, fix your thoughts on Jesus, whom we acknowledge as our apostle and high priest.
—Hebrews 3:1

Filling our minds with thoughts of Jesus is a great way to counteract discouragement and doubt. When we've had a setback and we're trying to get up on our feet again, thoughts of Jesus rising from the dead can give us hope. We can think about his tenderness in dealing with those in need, his bravery in facing suffering, his honesty, his wisdom, his strength. Whatever qualities we're lacking, we can tell God, "Please make me more like Jesus in this area of my life."

Jesus is our point of reference. How would Jesus approach a particular situation? What would give him the courage to do that? He is our standard of service, showing us how the King devotes himself to the needs of others. He demonstrates an eternal mindset, remembering that the most important things are those that will last beyond this life.

FOOD FOR THOUGHT

Jesus is God's messenger and the high priest who intercedes for us at the Father's throne.

MORNING SUPPORT

The Sovereign Lord has given me a well-instructed tongue, to know the word that sustains the weary. He wakens me morning by morning, wakens my ear to listen like one being instructed. —Isaiah 50:4

Isaiah had a habit of waking up in the morning and listening to God with a particular attitude: ready! He surrendered his day completely to God. Jesus had that same habit. The Bible says, "Very early in the morning, while it was still dark, Jesus got up, left the house and went off to a solitary place, where he prayed" (Mark 1:35).

Just as a good breakfast prepares us physically and mentally for the day, so a morning routine of time with God can transform us spiritually. It focuses our minds on what we most need to think about: God's agenda. It increases the likelihood that we will check in with God throughout the day. Isaiah said his habit equipped him to encourage tired people, and that will be true of us. When we've let God encourage and support us, we'll be in tune with God's desires for our day and much more equipped to support others.

FOOD FOR THOUGHT

Surrendering to God each morning is as nourishing for the spirit as a good breakfast is for the body.

THE FREEDOM OF SELF-CONTROL

The grace of God ... teaches us to say "No" to ungodliness and worldly passions, and to live self-controlled, upright and godly lives in this present age.
—Titus 2:11–12

We want to say no to unhealthy habits, but sometimes it's difficult, isn't it? Some habits can seem so deeply rooted that we aren't able to make good choices to break the unhealthy pattern.

What can we do? The Bible urges us to pray for the grace of God, which enables us to say no to unhealthy impulses and yes to self-controlled, upright, and godly habits. It turns out that self-control is true freedom, the freedom to choose what we know is good for us. We gain more self-control as we pray for grace and then act on grace. The more often we act on grace, the weaker the grip our old habits have on our lives. More and more, we'll be able to choose self-controlled practices.

FOOD FOR THOUGHT

Self-control is true freedom, and God's grace makes it available to us so we become fully free to make choices that will help us flourish.

IN THE FAMILY

For you know that it was not with perishable things such as silver or gold that you were redeemed from the empty way of life handed down to you from your ancestors, but with the precious blood of Christ, a lamb without blemish or defect. —1 Peter 1:18–19

God bought your freedom from an empty way of life at the price of the shed blood of his beloved Son. It's impossible to overstate how precious Jesus' life was, and yet he sacrificed it on your behalf. That's how much God cares about you.

God has adopted you as his own son or daughter, and he loves you immeasurably more than the best parent loves his child. God loves you the way he loves Jesus, his own Son.

Your worth comes from what Jesus did for you, not from your perfect performance. You may fall short on innumerable assignments from God, but he doesn't love you less for that. You "are counted as righteous, not because of [your] work, but because of [your] faith in God who forgives sinners" (Romans 4:5 NLT).

FOOD FOR THOUGHT

You were bought with the precious blood of Jesus; you're now God's child.

LISTENING TO GOD

"Listen to this, Job; stop and consider God's wonders."

—Job 37:14

If we want God to speak to us about his plans for our lives, we have to give him our undivided attention. He won't shout over the noise of the Internet, the television, our work, or our worries. We need unhurried time away from all of that so that we can listen.

Consider scheduling an uninterrupted morning for God. Get away from distractions. Turn off your phone. Ask God to help you screen out other voices—like your inner critic—that can compete for your attention. Use these precious hours to rest in God's presence, pour out your heart, and listen to his heart through his Word.

It may feel like you're far too busy to plan a block of time with God, but when else will you find the encouragement and guidance you need from the one who knows and loves you best?

FOOD FOR THOUGHT

God is longing to spend time with you to build you up, rejuvenate your soul, and show his wonders.

MORE OF GOD

You're blessed when you're at the end of your rope. With less of you there is more of God and his rule. —*Matthew 5:3 MSG*

Have you ever considered a setback as a blessing? First of all, setbacks aren't failures. They are the normal ups and downs of life. Second, God uses them to bring us to the end of our rope, the end of our own resources, so we learn to rely on his vast resources. Part of his design is for there to be less of us and more of him in our lives. John the Baptist said of Jesus, "He must become greater; I must become less" (John 3:30).

Surprisingly, when there is less of us and more of God, that's when we find ourselves most empowered to move forward. God says, "I live in a high and holy place, but also with the one who is contrite and lowly in spirit, to revive the spirit of the lowly and to revive the heart of the contrite" (Isaiah 57:15). So when a setback brings us low but we turn to God in that place, he'll get us back on our feet and running the marathon with joy.

FOOD FOR THOUGHT

Setbacks can be blessings, because when there's less of us, there's more of God and his rule, and that's where our true joy lies.

GENUINE

"I heard you in the garden, and I was afraid ... so I hid."

—*Genesis 3:10*

After Adam sinned for the first time, he felt an emotion he'd never felt before: shame. Shame makes us want to hide who we really are, because we believe we are defective and we don't want to be rejected. So when Adam felt shame and heard God coming, he hid.

We may not hide from people physically, but we do have all sorts of strategies for hiding emotionally. We wear masks that hide our needs and weaknesses to make people think we're smarter, stronger, and more together.

God did not give us a spirit of fear (2 Timothy 1:7). Instead he gave us his Holy Spirit who empowers us, whose love casts out fear, and who enables self-discipline. Whenever we find ourselves inclined to hide and fake it, we can call out for the Holy Spirit. Then we can be genuine with other people in the growth process we are all in, knowing each of us is a work in progress, unique and unfinished.

FOOD FOR THOUGHT

Let's be genuine in our relationships, because God loves us as we are and has given us a spirit of power and love.

THE END PRIZE

Everyone who competes in the games goes into strict training. They do it to get a crown that will not last, but we do it to get a crown that will last forever.
— *1 Corinthians 9:25*

In 1938, Károly Tákacs was the premier pistol shooter in the world, expected to win gold at the 1940 Olympics. But he was in the Hungarian army, and a live grenade exploded in his right hand, his shooting hand. For most people, that would have been the end of their Olympic hopes, but Tákacs was not most people.

For a year he trained to shoot with his left hand. He chose to focus not on his problem, but on the solution to it. Then he went to the 1939 World Championships—and won.

Once again, he was set up to compete in the 1940 Olympics. But the 1940 and 1944 games were cancelled because of World War II. So he waited until the 1948 Olympics, competed at last, and won the gold.[25]

Tákacs was focused on the prize. His eye was on his goal and what he needed to do to achieve it. We need that same focus. What do you want? What will it take to get there? Aim at a prize that will last forever.

FOOD FOR THOUGHT

God's glory and his pleasure are the prizes that will last forever; they are worth our full focus.

EXPOSING WHO YOU ARE

A bruised reed he will not break, and a smoldering wick he will not snuff out.
—Isaiah 42:3

Mutual vulnerability is a key feature of a true friendship. By definition, vulnerability means openness to emotional harm. No one wants to be harmed, so many people are afraid to be vulnerable. But if we have walls up against harm, we also have walls up against love. Until we let down those walls, we can't experience being deeply loved.

Isaiah prophesied that Jesus would be trustworthy with vulnerable people—those who are bruised and weary. We need to be like him in that trustworthiness, and we need friends who are similarly trustworthy. The truth is, in our deepest places we are all hurting and longing for love. Let's put away shame and break down walls, so others can come close to love us deeply.

Do you have one or two people in your life with whom you can safely be vulnerable? If you don't, consider taking a step of faith and being more honest with someone who seems trustworthy. Test the waters by calmly mentioning some area of weakness or need and seeing their response. It's definitely worth the risk.

FOOD FOR THOUGHT

People who offer the precious gift of trustworthiness will help you feel loved and secure in your vulnerability.

IN DEEP WATER

When you pass through the waters, I will be with you; and when you pass through the rivers, they will not sweep over you. When you walk through the fire, you will not be burned; the flames will not set you ablaze.

—*Isaiah 43:2*

Sometimes change feels like wading through a rushing river. But God promises he will not allow you to drown. God is with you, whether you feel it or not. Feelings aren't a reliable gauge of his presence. He will walk next to you and help you deal with whatever you're going through.

Moses told God, "If your Presence does not go with us, do not send us up from here" (Exodus 33:15). He knew the Israelites couldn't accomplish their mission without God's presence and help. God reassured Moses that he would absolutely go with them, and he kept that promise.

Step forward, confident in God's help that's only a prayer away.

FOOD FOR THOUGHT

God will make sure you get safely to the other side; he will be faithful to sustain you and put you on dry ground again.

QUIETNESS AND CONFIDENCE

"In repentance and rest is your salvation, in quietness and trust is your strength."

—Isaiah 30:15

Strength is not found in frantic activity but in resting in the stillness of God's presence. In these moments, we can let his love permeate our hearts. We can let the radiance of his glory shine on us. We can refocus our thoughts from our problems to the greatness of God.

We need times when we draw quietly into his presence and simply worship him for being God. He invites us to cultivate a practice of carving out moments of stillness, of practicing rest, of sitting before him without an agenda.

God rarely shouts. Most of the time he speaks to us quietly. And we are most receptive to input when we are quiet. Further, while change does require effort on our part, it just as often requires the skill of relinquishing control to God, trusting his plans and his ways. That skill is best learned when we're restful. For all these reasons, quietness is always a good friend.

FOOD FOR THOUGHT

A quiet heart is open to God and open to the change he offers.

EXTRAVAGANT LOVE

This is how God showed his love among us: He sent his one and only Son into the world that we might live through him. This is love: not that we loved God, but that he loved us and sent his Son as an atoning sacrifice for our sins. —1 John 4:9–10

Sometimes our minds get hazy about how much God loves us. Maybe we've had a yo-yo experience of going up and down with our weight or a chronic health issue or our fitness goals, and deep down we feel that God's love is based on how we're performing in a particular area. When those feelings arise, we need to go back to the basics.

God showed how much he loves us by sending his one and only Son into the world to die for us. God delights in us with an extravagant love that is beyond our comprehension. We need to build our lives on the foundation of God's ongoing love that sacrifices everything for us. That's real love that never gives up on us, no matter what.

FOOD FOR THOUGHT

"How glorious the splendor of a human heart which trusts that it is loved." —Brennan Manning[26]

GOD WILL FINISH IT

I am certain that God, who began the good work within you, will continue his work until it is finally finished on the day when Christ Jesus returns.
—*Philippians 1:6 NLT*

You cannot reach your goals by human willpower alone. The apostle Paul says, "It is God who works in you to will and to act in order to fulfill his good purpose" (Philippians 2:13). Both the desire and the power come ultimately from God, but you need to consciously depend on him for these two things, asking for them regularly.

You didn't begin the good work within you; God did. And God will keep right on helping you grow in his grace until his purpose for you is fulfilled.

Focus on Christ. Don't focus on your failures. Failures are simply an opportunity to learn. When things don't go your way, when you get frustrated, look to God's strength and resist discouragement. If necessary, make a U-turn and start again. Keep relying on Christ. He won't give up.

FOOD FOR THOUGHT

God longs to show himself as faithful. He promises to complete that good work within you.

RESTFUL

*Whoever dwells in the shelter of the Most High will rest in the shadow of
the Almighty. I will say of the Lord, "He is my refuge and my fortress, my
God, in whom I trust."* —Psalm 91:1–2

The Daniel Plan's Five Essentials work together so that we are
nourished spiritually, physically, mentally, and emotionally.
Part of that nourishment comes from the rest and restoration of our
bodies, minds, and souls. How glorious is the rest and restoration we
have when we come to God!

The psalmist says God is our refuge, our place of safety, the one
who gives us rest. He goes on to say, "under his wings you will find
refuge" (91:4). When we're feeling vulnerable, we can actually hide
under God's wings and know we're safe and loved there.

Deuteronomy 33:12 offers a similar promise: "Let the beloved of
the LORD rest secure in him, for he shields him all day long, and the
one the LORD loves rests between his shoulders." Do you need rest
today? Run to God and accept what he freely offers.

FOOD FOR THOUGHT

Whenever we're running on empty, we can go to God
and find rest, refuge, and safety.

A STEP OF FAITH

Moses said to God, "Who am I that I should go to Pharaoh and bring the Israelites out of Egypt?" And God said, "I will be with you."

—Exodus 3:11–12

Moses felt inadequate. He didn't know how to speak well in public. He thought he was no match for the king of Egypt. But God said he would make up for Moses' inadequacy.

God gave Moses the power to do several miraculous things, and Moses still asked God to send someone else. Finally God said, "See that you perform before Pharaoh all the wonders I have given you the power to do" (Exodus 4:21).

We can relate to Moses' feelings of inadequacy. We know we're not the person who will always hit a homerun. We don't always feel equipped, and yet God calls us to step out in faith anyway. Life in Christ isn't about our perfect performance; it's about the power of a surrendered life. God says, "See that you do all I have given you the power to do." Will you trust him and go?

FOOD FOR THOUGHT

It's not about our adequacy; it's about God's.

HOPE FOR THE HARVEST

Let's not get tired of doing what is good. At just the right time we will reap a harvest of blessing if we don't give up. —*Galatians 6:9 NLT*

We all get physically tired and need rest. But the apostle Paul urges us not to get emotionally and spiritually tired of doing good. We need to hold on to the hope that doing what is right will lead to a harvest of blessing.

Sometimes we falter in doing good because of sin or fatigue. Sometimes we falter because of pressure. Sometimes we falter because doing good takes extra effort. But if we muster the courage to stand up and do what is right, in the long run the result will be a harvest of blessing. We need the stamina that comes from a long habit of doing good. When we practice doing good in small ways over and over, it builds up a powerful habit to do good even when it's tough.

Perhaps there is someone you can encourage today, some small step of kindness you can take, or a ministry you can participate in that pours life into others. Whatever it is, know that you are investing in a habit that will result in good for you and for many.

FOOD FOR THOUGHT

Doing good leads to more good, as others pass on what they have received from us.

A WAY OUT

No test or temptation that comes your way is beyond the course of what others have had to face. . . . God will never let you down; he'll never let you be pushed past your limit; he'll always be there to help you come through it.
—*1 Corinthians 10:13 MSG*

We're all tempted. It's part of being human. The Bible says even Jesus was tempted. It's not a sin to be tempted. It's more like, "Welcome to the human race."

No matter what temptation we face, others have faced that same temptation. Some days we give in, while on other days we are able to resist. But God promises he will always provide a means of escape. We won't have to search for it or feel helpless. He shows us the way. What a fantastic promise this is: God will always provide a way out. That is grace! We can simply turn the channel, or run out the door, or change the way we're thinking. There's always grace to get through.

FOOD FOR THOUGHT

When we're tempted, it's just part of growth. And as we look to God, he will provide a way out.

UNFORGETTABLE

See, I have engraved you on the palms of my hands.

—*Isaiah 49:16*

God is greater than the universe, and yet he's close to each one of us. He sees you, and he knows everything about you, including the areas where you feel stuck and the areas where you want to grow. He has engraved you on the palms of his hand, where Jesus bears the wounds of his crucifixion. "Even the very hairs of your head are all numbered" (Matthew 10:30).

Growth comes as we become more grounded in the faith that God has this kind of love for us. As Paul prayed, "Christ will make his home in your hearts as you trust in him. Your roots will grow down into God's love and keep you strong. And may you have the power to understand, as all God's people should, how wide, how long, how high, and how deep his love is. May you experience the love of Christ, though it is too great to understand fully. Then you will be made complete with all the fullness of life and power that comes from God" (Ephesians 3:17–20 NLT).

FOOD FOR THOUGHT

The great, almighty God who rules the universe also loves and cares for each one of us.

LOOKING BEYOND

Now is your time of grief, but I will see you again and you will rejoice, and no one will take away your joy. —*John 16:22*

Hours before he was arrested and killed, Jesus promised his followers that they would have a temporary time of grief (when all seemed lost) and then a permanent time of joy (when he rose from the dead). The same is true for us. When we suffer a tragedy or a delay in seeing God work in our lives, or we hit a wall, grief can feel overwhelming. And yet God promises joy will come. In times like these, we need to cling to his promises. We need to remember what God has shown us in the light.

Even when it's hard to envision life beyond grief, God has a plan in motion and always offers his presence as assurance. In the midst of our pain, we can invite God to make room in our hearts so bitterness has no room to grow. We make suffering an open invitation for God to work in us.

The Bible says, "Blessed is the one who trusts in the LORD, whose confidence is in him. They will be like a tree planted by the water that sends out its roots by the stream. It does not fear when heat comes; its leaves are always green" (Jeremiah 17:7–8).

FOOD FOR THOUGHT

No matter what we suffer, God's presence will always be with us, and he will bring us back to joy.

SEE AND HEAR

The LORD make his face shine on you and be gracious to you.
—Numbers 6:25

Our prayer is that the Lord will make his face shine on us and be gracious to us. Yet sometimes it's hard to see his graciousness in our lives because we get busy or overwhelmed by circumstances. We need to slow down so we can see that grace is everywhere.

Frederick Buechner said, "Listen to your life. See it for the fathomless mystery it is. In the boredom and pain of it, no less than in the excitement and gladness: touch, taste, smell your way to the holy and hidden heart of it, because in the last analysis all moments are key moments, and life itself is grace."[27]

We need to be intentional in listening and seeing. We put ourselves in a mode of gratitude, which always opens our eyes and ears to God's face shining on us, giving us improbable moments of grace. His presence, his power, his peace are there to be heard as we listen closely.

FOOD FOR THOUGHT

When we slow down to listen, we will see and hear his overflowing graciousness.

EXPECT TO FALL

Even if godly people fall down seven times, they always get up.
—*Proverbs 24:16 NIrV*

E ven good people stumble. Even people who are trying to do what's right make mistakes. We're bound to be imperfect in following The Daniel Plan. Successful people aren't those who never fail. They're those who refuse to quit.

Paul was a good example of this. He says, "We are hard pressed on every side, but not crushed; perplexed, but not in despair; persecuted, but not abandoned; struck down, but not destroyed" (2 Corinthians 4:8–9).

Great people are simply ordinary people with extraordinary determination. They know they're never a failure, and the main goal is to get up again after a bad day or a bad season.

God is not waiting for you to get physically healthy or spiritually mature before he starts loving you and enjoying you. He loves you right now. He is not waiting for you to cross the finish line first. He is smiling at you as you run the race. And if you stumble, he cheers even more loudly to encourage you to stand up again.

FOOD FOR THOUGHT

We're all in this race together, running imperfectly but not giving up, as God roots for us to go the next leg of the race.

GOD CHOSE YOU

God chose us to belong to Christ before the world was created. He chose us to be holy and without blame in his eyes. He loved us.

—Ephesians 1:4 NIrV

God chose you before he made the oceans. Before he made the solar system, before the sun burst into existence. Before he spread the galaxies of stars across the universe. Before all that, he decided he was going to choose to love you. "Once you were not a people, but now you are the people of God; once you had not received mercy, but now you have received mercy" (1 Peter 2:10).

If God put so much into creating you, why would you want to be anyone else?

It's so important to be secure in your identity as one of God's very own. In order to move forward and make all the changes you desire on The Daniel Plan, you need to know at a profound level how much God loves you. That will radically change your motivation.

FOOD FOR THOUGHT

God says he chose you from the very start; you are part of his family. In his eyes you are holy and without fault.

GOD IS TRUSTWORTHY

When I am afraid, I put my trust in you. In God, whose word I praise—
in God I trust and am not afraid. What can mere mortals do to me?

—Psalm 56:3–4

The chief response God is looking for as we face any circumstance is trust. The Bible says we can trust that his word is true. We can trust that his promises are real, that he wrote them for us. We can trust that all things are possible with God. That nothing is too difficult for him, that his strength is shown in our weakness, that his grace is sufficient for us. We can count on these things.

Isaiah says to God, "You will keep in perfect peace those whose minds are steadfast, because they trust in you. Trust in the LORD forever, for the LORD, the LORD himself, is the Rock eternal" (Isaiah 26:3–4). What an amazing promise: we will have perfect peace if we can put fear aside and trust God's good plan for our lives.

FOOD FOR THOUGHT

God is absolutely trustworthy and anything is possible for him, even things we hardly dare to dream of.

EVERY PART OF YOU

*Offer yourselves to God as those who have been brought from death to life;
and offer every part of yourself to him as an instrument of righteousness.*
—Romans 6:13

God has given us so much. He enables us to see, hear, breathe. In Jesus' resurrection he has brought us back from death too. He wants every part of us to be a tool in his hands for good purposes. But we often hold certain pieces of ourselves back.

God is doing so many things right now that are bigger than our problems. God has a much bigger picture in mind, and he wants us to be part of it. What are you holding back? Will you give every part of who you are to God's work? We have the privilege of being tools in his hands. The Bible says we are "created in Christ Jesus to do good works, which God prepared in advance for us to do" (Ephesians 2:10).

FOOD FOR THOUGHT

God has good purposes for us and wants to use everything about us to help change the world.

GOD'S FAITHFULNESS

The LORD is trustworthy in all he promises and faithful in all he does.
—Psalm 145:13

God is faithful. That is, he is persistently loyal, offers constant support, and keeps his promises to those he has brought into his family. He is consistent and reliable. In fact, the Bible tells us that even "if we are faithless, he remains faithful, for he cannot disown himself" (2 Timothy 2:13). Even if we are disloyal to him, he doesn't respond in kind. His faithfulness depends on his own unchanging character, not on our perfect behavior.

This is so important for us, because as we pursue growth in The Daniel Plan, we will have imperfect performance. We may have days when we doubt God, when we want to quit—and even days when we do quit. Fortunately, God remains faithful to us, urging us to start again, providing the strength we need to renew our hope. His love and his help remain constant.

FOOD FOR THOUGHT

We can return to God again and again, trusting that he is unfailingly faithful no matter what.

PERSEVERANCE IN OPPOSITION

Then Joshua son of Jozadak and his fellow priests and Zerubbabel son of Shealtiel and his associates began to build the altar of the God of Israel to sacrifice burnt offerings on it.... Despite their fear of the peoples around them, they built the altar on its foundation. —Ezra 3:2–3

After seventy years of exile, a remnant of Jews got permission from the king of Persia to return to Judah. They were led by the priest Joshua and Zerubbabel, a descendant of King David. These two men led those who shared a big dream: to rebuild the temple in Jerusalem and to re-establish the nation of God's people.

They faced great opposition, especially from the non-Jews who had settled the land in their absence. Despite their fear of those people, they built an altar on the temple site to make offerings to God.

If you face opposition as you seek to reach your goals and fulfill your dreams, take courage from the example of Joshua and Zerubbabel, who persevered and eventually led the remnant to rebuild a temple. God was with them, and he enabled them far beyond anything they could do on their own.

FOOD FOR THOUGHT

God is with you, enabling you to reach your goals for your blessing and his own glory.

UNFAILING LOVE

But I trust in your unfailing love; my heart rejoices in your salvation.
—*Psalm 13:5*

Unfailing love is a key feature of God's character. The Hebrew word translated as unfailing love reflects an enduring commitment because of a personal relationship. God's love doesn't come and go on the whims of emotion. It is reliable. Also, he expresses it through action, not just words. God constantly treats us with unfailing love, and he will never fail to do so.

He wants us to depend on his unfailing love. Our hope rests not on our own strength but on his reliable, committed care for us. When we call out to him to deliver us, we can expect a response because of his loving nature. When we have setbacks and fail to perform as well as we'd like, his love yet again doesn't waver. He who demonstrated his unfailing love on the cross will certainly stand with us as we seek to grow in faith.

FOOD FOR THOUGHT

God's love endures forever; it is faithful, true, and sure.

POURING FORTH KINDNESS

But the fruit of the Spirit is love, joy, peace, forbearance, kindness, goodness, faithfulness, gentleness and self-control. —Galatians 5:22–23

Kindness is one proof of the Holy Spirit's work in us. The more we give free rein to the Spirit to transform our hearts, the more we will overflow with kindness toward ourselves and others.

It's common to have an inner critic that speaks harshly about our body or our performance. As we grow in kindness, the voice of that inner critic will gradually decrease and a voice of kind encouragement will get easier to hear. The encouraging voice says that our bodies are temples of the Holy Spirit and beloved by God. It says we are dearly loved regardless of our performance.

The Bible says, "Therefore, as God's chosen people, holy and dearly loved, clothe yourselves with compassion, kindness, humility, gentleness and patience" (Colossians 3:12). As we know more and more that we are dearly loved, kindness will grow. As the Spirit fosters kindness in us, we will look for ways to help others live well. What opportunity for kindness do you have today?

FOOD FOR THOUGHT

Let the fruit of kindness grow in your heart and in your interactions with others.

SEEING CLEARLY

Your eye is the lamp of your body. When your eyes are healthy, your whole body also is full of light. But when they are unhealthy, your body also is full of darkness.
—Luke 11:34

When Jesus speaks here about our eyes, he isn't talking about physical eyesight, whether we need contact lenses or cataract surgery. He's talking about the eyes of our minds, what we focus on. For each one of us, our minds create a pair of glasses through which we see the world. If those glasses are good, then we see things clearly. If they're bad, we see everything in a distorted way. So in order to have a healthy life, we need to attend to the direction of our thoughts. Where do our minds go automatically?

Pastor Rick Warren says, "The battle starts not in your belly; it starts in your brain." Throughout the day, pay attention to where your mind goes. When you think about food or fitness or the goals you're setting for your life, how do you think about them? Do you see them through a negative filter, or do you have eyes that help you see things as they really are?

FOOD FOR THOUGHT

If the eyes of your mind are healthy, your whole being will be full of light, and you'll be able to see everything clearly.

LIFE THROUGH THE WORD

Turn your ear to my words. Do not let them out of your sight, keep them within your heart; for they are life to those who find them and health to one's whole body. —Proverbs 4:20–22

If we want to be healthy, we need to let the words in the Bible penetrate deeply into our hearts. We need to learn how to listen carefully to them, to spend enough time with them that we really hear them. If we do that, they will bring life and healing to us. Real life is found nowhere else.

God says, "Don't lose sight of them." This is a matter of mental focus. It's easy for the busyness of the day to drive out the memory of what we heard in God's Word. On the other hand, taking a moment to recall a verse can make a big difference in how his words influence us. What was it that God said? How is it relevant here and now, in this moment?

The more time we spend in God's Word, the more we fill our minds with light and life, and the healthier we will be.

FOOD FOR THOUGHT

The more we immerse ourselves in the words of Scripture, the more life and health we will have.

WITH WINGS

Even youths grow tired and weary, and young men stumble and fall; but those who hope in the Lord will renew their strength. They will soar on wings like eagles; they will run and not grow weary, they will walk and not be faint. —Isaiah 40:30–31

Discouragement weighs us down; hope lifts us up and gets us going. If we want more energy, the Bible says to put hope in the Lord. Those who place their confident expectation in God will boost their power. They will soar and run without tiring out.

Hope is something we choose to foster by feeding on God's Word. We can feed hope or we can feed discouragement, depending on what we choose to think about.

When we hope in the Lord, we won't be disappointed. The psalmist says to God, "No one who hopes in you will ever be put to shame" (Psalm 25:3). We can confidently look forward to God fulfilling every word he has promised.

FOOD FOR THOUGHT

We are strong, energized, and encouraged when God is the focus of our hope.

GOD-DEPENDENT

Ah, Sovereign LORD, you have made the heavens and the earth by your
great power and outstretched arm. Nothing is too hard for you.
—Jeremiah 32:17

God spoke all things into being, and he sustains all things—every cell, every star, every thought. We cannot think up anything that would be impossible for him to do.

His name the LORD in Hebrew means *he is*. It's related to his name for himself: I AM. He exists by his own power; everything else exists by dependence on him. I AM also implies *I am actively present*. He's not far away in a distant heaven; he's right here, as close as your breath.

This is the God you are trusting to get you to the finish line. He sustains galaxies, and he can certainly sustain you. What do you need from our all-powerful God?

FOOD FOR THOUGHT

As we meditate on the power it takes to hold all the stars in the universe in place and keep the earth spinning at the right speed, we have some glimpse of the awesome power God has to work in our lives.

PERFECT GOODNESS

You are good and what you do is good; teach me your decrees.

—Psalm 119:68

God is perfectly good, and everything he does is good. In fact, he is the standard by which we know what good is.

Sometimes we don't understand why he allows difficult circumstances in our lives. "How could a good God allow this?" we ask. But even when he doesn't explain himself, we can be confident that his heart is good toward us. He wants to bring good out of every circumstance, even the most painful.

The place where we see the goodness of God most clearly is on the cross. He entered our world and experienced the worst suffering for our sakes. He brought good out of evil human choices to show us that he can and will bring good out of anything.

FOOD FOR THOUGHT

We can be absolutely confident that God always has good at heart. He will bring good out of whatever we're going through.

IMMANUEL

The virgin will conceive and give birth to a son, and they will call him
Immanuel (which means "God with us").   —Matthew 1:23

The prophet Isaiah predicted that a child named Immanuel would be born as a sign of God's power and presence with his people (Isaiah 7:14). Seven centuries later, Jesus was born of a virgin, and one of the names the Bible gives him is Immanuel, which means *God with us.*

Jesus is fully God, and he became a mortal man to take on everything we experience. He became human to show us that God is not far away in heaven, indifferent to what we're going through, but is in fact *God with us* every moment.

As you take this journey toward health, call out to him as Immanuel. He is with you, and he cares about what you're going through. He has experienced every aspect of human life that you will go through. He is with you every step of the way.

FOOD FOR THOUGHT

Jesus is God with us at every moment, encouraging and strengthening us to keep pursuing this adventure of being fully his.

WHAT GETS YOUR ATTENTION?

Absalom behaved in this way toward all the Israelites who came to the king asking for justice, and so he stole the hearts of the people of Israel.

—2 Samuel 15:6

Whatever gets your attention gets you. We can see that at work in the story of Absalom, son of King David. Absalom was angry at his father, because David hadn't punished Absalom's half-brother for abusing his sister. Absalom took revenge on the half-brother, but his anger didn't end there. He decided to win the people's support for a coup that sent David into exile and put Absalom on the throne. He humiliated his father in every way he could find. His efforts caused a civil war that ended in his own violent death.

Absalom became tragically fixated on one idea: the desire for revenge. We, too, can become fixated on unhealthy ideas and emotions. But we're not helpless. The choice to change what we focus on is always before us. God asks if we will decide to forgive or think about what is good, true, and noble. We can decide to meditate on Scripture. And when we do that, what gets our attention gets us for the better.

FOOD FOR THOUGHT

God gives us the power to focus our attention on goodness, truth, and forgiveness.

NEW WORK

See, the former things have taken place, and new things I declare; before they spring into being I announce them to you."　　　—*Isaiah 42:9*

God loves doing something new—that's his great pleasure! He has plans for our lives, and he'll let us in on them step by step when we're ready to know. We need to move forward into the next step in God's plan for us with eagerness even when he doesn't reveal what's beyond it. The Bible says, "This resurrection life you received from God is not a timid, grave-tending life. It's adventurously expectant, greeting God with a childlike 'What's next, Papa?'" (Romans 8:15 MSG).

What is the new thing God is focused on in your life today? Is he drawing you into a new way of eating? More movement throughout your day? Deepening your faith? Teaming up with some new friends? Replacing toxic thoughts with true ones? Don't be shy about moving forward into his new plan for you. Every step of the way, God has good intentions at heart.

FOOD FOR THOUGHT

The new thing God is doing in your life will help you flourish, and you can move into it with confidence.

PROGRESS NOT PERFECTION

From now on I will tell you about new things that will happen. I have not made them known to you before. —Isaiah 48:6 NIrV

When we begin any new habit, our performance is bound to be imperfect. Usually, for a while, we jostle between the new ways and the old ways. The new ways are unfamiliar; they take getting used to. That's why in The Daniel Plan we talk about progress, not perfection.

God's amazing grace is not just that he forgives our failures, but he also gives us the power to start over. He promises that he will fit everything, even our setbacks and relapses, into his plan and purpose for our lives. When we get off track, we simply stop, make a U-turn, and get back on the right road. We pray, "Lord, please bring us back to you. Then we can return. Make our lives like new again" (Lamentations 5:21 NIrV). The wonder of his grace is that he gives us that fresh start again and again, as many times as it takes.

FOOD FOR THOUGHT

As you're learning a new way of living, you get as many chances as it takes to keep starting afresh.

VIEW OF THE ALMIGHTY

"I am El-Shaddai—'God Almighty.' Serve me faithfully and live a blameless life."   *—Genesis 17:1 NLT*

One of God's names is God Almighty, or *El-Shaddai* in Hebrew. The root meaning of *El* is power. The root meaning of *Shaddai* is sufficiency and nourishment. God has ultimate power, and he uses it to nourish his people as a mother feeds an infant. He is sufficient for all our needs.

God says, "Can a mother forget the baby at her breast and have no compassion on the child she has borne? Though she may forget, I will not forget you!" (Isaiah 49:15). The all-powerful God is even more attentive to our needs than a mother is. He always remembers us.

As we're making changes, it's important to keep these truths about God at the forefront of our minds. The way we think determines the way we feel, and what we feel determines what we do. This is especially true of the way we think about God. He's right here with us, completely sufficient, providing what we need to change.

FOOD FOR THOUGHT

God is El-Shaddai, the Almighty, the All-Sufficient, the nourisher of our bodies and souls.

LIKE A SHEPHERD

Hear us, Shepherd of Israel, you who lead Joseph like a flock.

—Psalm 80:1

The job of a shepherd in ancient Israel was to keep his flock alive. He protected his sheep from lions and wolves. He made sure they had good grass and water even in areas that were semi-desert. If a sheep wandered off and got lost or fell and couldn't get up, the shepherd went searching for the sheep and restored it to safety. All of this nurturing and protecting was in King David's mind when he said, "The Lord is my shepherd" (Psalm 23:1).

God is committed to our well-being. Though many challenges can befall us, we can call on him to defend us and bring us through. We can ask him to provide what we need to nourish our bodies and souls. He wants to lead us to safety, and that means we need to follow him as attentively as sheep follow their shepherd. And even if we wander off course, he promises to guide us back to the right path.

FOOD FOR THOUGHT

God is the Shepherd; he will lead us on the road to still waters and green pastures that will restore our body and spirit.

CALL ON HIM

The Lord is near to all who call on him, to all who call on him in truth.
—Psalm 145:18

When we're tempted to get discouraged, it's important to know that the Lord is near to all who call on him. He's not far away and busy; he's near. He wants to hear from us. He wants us to call on him with our needs.

Pastor Rick Warren says, "You get the power to keep going from God, by asking him to empower you, and trusting in him moment by moment." Asking is important; it's one of the ways we cooperate with him in pursuing the goals he has for us. God wants us to have a relationship with him, and asking for his help is a way of saying, "I need you. Please be involved in my life."

The psalms are full of passionate prayers calling on God for help. "Since you are my rock and my fortress, for the sake of your name lead and guide me" (Psalm 31:3). "Keep me safe, O God, I've run for dear life to you. I say to God, 'Be my Lord!' Without you, nothing makes sense" (Psalm 16:1–2 MSG). These are models for us to follow.

FOOD FOR THOUGHT

Calling upon God with confidence deepens our relationship with him; he will always respond and renew us.

YOUR WORK

As each part does its own special work, it helps the other parts grow, so that the whole body is healthy and growing and full of love.

—*Ephesians 4:16 NLT*

You were designed to get healthy in partnership with others. The Christian community is a body. The whole body gets healthy and full of love when each part does its own job, helping the other parts grow. You have something to contribute to the growth and health of others, and you need them to help you grow. In fact, you won't grow as much without working with others.

Who are the people who really know you, who care what you're going through? Who are the people you really know and care about? Loving others is meant to be one of your top priorities. It's essential for serving God and improving your health. Engage in this marvelous adventure of investing in others' lives and letting them invest in yours, so that ultimately Christ's whole body is healthy and full of love.

FOOD FOR THOUGHT

Reap the huge benefits of interdependence with others in your journey toward health.

RELIABLE COMFORTER

Why, my soul, are you downcast? Why so disturbed within me? Put your hope in God, for I will yet praise him, my Savior and my God.

—*Psalm 42:5*

There will inevitably be times when your soul is downcast. But if you put your hope in God, you won't stay there for long. God is high and holy, yet he doesn't stay far off in that high and holy place, distant from us and our needs. If you're low-spirited because you've had a setback in pursuing your health goals, God is right there with you. He doesn't just visit the downcast, he moves in and camps alongside you. He is committed to helping you get up and on your feet again.

The Bible says, "Cast your cares on the Lord and he will sustain you; he will never let the righteous be shaken" (Psalm 55:22). That's a promise you can count on. God wants to carry your load with you. What do you need to pile onto his shoulders? God will live with you and help you through your challenges.

FOOD FOR THOUGHT

Put your hope in God; he is the most reliable comforter. You can depend on him.

BECOMING HOLY

Keep my decrees and follow them. I am the LORD, who makes you holy.
—*Leviticus 20:8*

One of God's names in the Old Testament is Yahweh-M'Kaddesh, the Lord who makes you holy. This name speaks to our desire to become more and more like Christ as his power works in and through us. "God planned that those he had chosen would become like his Son. In that way, Christ will be the first and most honored among many brothers and sisters" (Romans 8:29 NIrV).

Becoming like Christ takes effort on our part in partnership with the Holy Spirit. We choose to spend time alone with him, soaking in his holiness. We choose to let him shine his spotlight on our lives, illuminating areas where he wants to change our habits. We choose to step out in faith, relying on the Spirit's power to enable us to do what we couldn't do on our own. Gradually, the new way becomes familiar, as natural as walking but walking in his ways.

FOOD FOR THOUGHT

God gives us the privilege of becoming more and more like Christ every day.

GOD'S PROVISION

*And my God will meet all your needs according to the riches of his glory in
Christ Jesus.* —Philippians 4:19

God provides everything we need, not sparingly but according
to his riches. He provides for us spiritually, sending friends to
care for us and his Word to feed our souls. He also provides for us
physically. Think about the abundance of foods he has made available
to us; your local grocery store probably has dozens of fruits and vegetables, as well as a variety of nuts, whole grains, dried beans, herbs,
and spices. If you visit ethnic grocery stores, you'll find flavorful new
mushrooms, salty sea vegetables, and other plants you never dreamed
of. Ultimately, all food comes from God as he works through the array
of growers and markets to take it from the field to our tables.

He promises, "Those who seek the LORD lack no good thing"
(Psalm 34:10). Treat God's provision as an adventure. Lay your needs
before him and watch him provide.

FOOD FOR THOUGHT

We can be confident of always having enough good
things to nourish us, because God provides generously.

YESTERDAY, TODAY, AND TOMORROW

My mouth will tell of your righteous deeds, of your saving acts all day long.
—*Psalm 71:15*

Pastor Rick Warren says, "Remind yourself of God's goodness yesterday, God's presence today, God's promises for tomorrow." If we want reassurance that he is perfectly good, perfectly wise, and all-powerful, the Bible vividly recounts his righteous deeds and saving acts, his mighty acts of goodness.

We also need to remind ourselves of God's goodness to us personally then and now. How have you experienced his goodness in your life? What would happen if you kept a record of all the glorious things God does for you, so you could look back at it when you need encouragement? The psalmist says to God, "You know when I sit and when I rise; you perceive my thoughts from afar" (Psalm 139:2). He says God is there with him wherever he goes.

Finally, we remind ourselves of his promises for tomorrow, such as "'Because he loves me,' says the LORD, 'I will rescue him; I will protect him, for he acknowledges my name'" (Psalm 91:14).

FOOD FOR THOUGHT

Remembering what God has done, thanking him for what he is doing, and hoping in what he is going to do will keep our hearts and minds steadfast.

ALL YOUR HEART

Whatever you do, work at it with all your heart, as working for the Lord, not for human masters. —*Colossians 3:23*

What motivates you to get healthy? It's completely legitimate to do it out of love for someone else, such as your spouse or your grandkids. It's also legitimate to do it for yourself, so that you feel better or are able to participate in activities that require energy and focus. Many other motivations are equally valid and lead to numerous rewards for pursuing health.

God gives you all these incentives to get healthy, but he also has one more he would like you to consider. Do it for him. It's a great energizer if you decide that all the work of getting healthy is ultimately not for anyone but the Lord. That's a motivation that can help you move through whatever setbacks come your way. As the apostle Paul said, "So whether you eat or drink or whatever you do, do it all for the glory of God" (1 Corinthians 10:31).

FOOD FOR THOUGHT

Pursue your goals with all your heart, and whatever your other motivations, do it ultimately for the Lord.

NOTES

1. Frederick Buechner, *Beyond Words* (San Francisco: HarperOne, 2004), 413.

2. Barbara Bradley Hagerty, "Prayer May Reshape Your Brain ... And Your Reality," NPR, May 20, 2009, http://www.npr.org/templates/story/story .php?storyId=104310443.

3. "Brennan Manning on Ruthless Trust," *Christianity Today*, Dec. 1, 2002, http://www.christianitytoday.com/ct/2002/decemberweb-only/ 12-9-21.0.html.

4. L. Stahre and T. Hallstrom, "A short-term cognitive group treatment program ... ," *Eating and Weight Disorders*, (March 2005): 51–58; Ruth Streigel-Moore, G. Terence Wilson, et al. "Cognitive behavioral guided self-help ... ," *Journal of Consulting and Clinical Psychology* (June 2010).

5. Charles Spurgeon, "Trials," *3-Minute Devotions with Charles Spurgeon*, (Uhrichsville, OH: Barbour Publishing, 2015), 56.

6. Tim Funk, "Q&A: Billy Graham at 90," *Christianity Today*, Nov. 7, 2008, http://www.christianitytoday.com/ct/2008/novemberweb-only/145-52 .0.html.

7. "Choosing Faith over Fear," *In Touch*, Aug. 22, 2014, http://www.oneplace .com/devotionals/in-touch-with-charles-stanley/in-touch-august-22-2013 -11675920.html.

8. "Mother Theresa: Her Own Words," Mother Theresa of Calcutta Center, mothertheresa.org, http://www.mothertheresa.org/layout.html.

9. Eugene H. Peterson, *A Long Obedience in the Same Direction: Discipleship in an Instant Society* (Downers Grove, IL: InterVarsity, 1980), 13.

10. Erika Andersen, "21 Quotes From Henry Ford On Business, Leadership And Life," Forbes.com, http://www.forbes.com/sites/erikaandersen/ 2013/05/31/21-quotes-from-henry-ford-on-business-leadership-and-life/.

11. "Henri Nouwen," L'Arche USA, http://www.larcheusa.org/learn/ henri-nouwen/.

12. Fraser Cain, "How Long Will Life Survive On Earth," Universetoday.com (Sept. 30, 2013), http://www.universetoday.com/25367/how-long-will -life-survive-on-earth/.

13. Corrie Ten Boom, *The Hiding Place* (Peabody, MA: Hendrickson Publishers, Inc., 2006), 240.

14. Viktor E. Frankl, *Man's Search for Meaning* (New York: Touchstone, 1984), 61.

15. "In Praise of Gratitude," Harvard Mental Health Newsletter (Nov. 2011), http://www.health.harvard.edu/newsletters/ Harvard_Mental_Health_Letter/2011/November/in-praise-of-gratitude

16. Billy Graham, *Nearing Home: Life, Faith and Finishing Well*, (Nashville: Thomas Nelson, 2011), 95.

17. Henri Nouwen, *Out of Solitude* (Notre Dame, IN: Ave Maria Press, 2004).

18. Brennan Manning, *The Ragamuffin Gospel* (Sisters, OR: Multnomah, 2000), 26.

19. Brennan Manning, *Abba's Child* (Colorado Springs, CO: NavPress, 2015), 42.

20. "Brennan Manning on Ruthless Trust," *Christianity Today* (Dec. 1, 2002), http://www.christianitytoday.com/ct/2002/decemberweb-only/12-9 -21.0.html.

21. Cornelius Plantinga Jr., *Not the Way It's Supposed to Be* (Grand Rapids: William B. Eerdmans Publishing Co., 1995), 10.

22. Henri Nouwen, *Life of the Beloved*, (Danvers, MA: The Crossroad Publishing Co., 2002), 59.

23. C.H. Spurgeon, The Metropolitan Tabernacle Pulpit: Sermons, parts 381392, (London: Passamore & Alabaster, 1887), 267.

24. Graham, *Nearing Home: Life, Faith and Finishing Well*, 95.

25. "Károly Tákacs Medals," Olympic.org, http://www.olympic.org/karoly -takacs.

26. Brennan Manning, *Ruthless Trust: The Ragamuffin's Path to God* (New York: HarperCollins, 2000), 148.

27. Frederick Buechner, "Listen to Your Life," Frederickbuchner.com, http:// frederickbuechner.com/content/listen-your-life.

≡✝DANIELPLAN

The Daniel Plan

40 Days to a Healthier Life

Rick Warren D. Min., Daniel Amen M.D., Mark Hyman M.D.

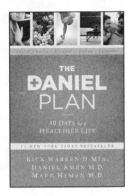

Revolutionizing The Concept of a Healthy Lifestyle

God designed our bodies to be healthy, providing everything we need to thrive and live abundantly. And with assistance from medical and fitness experts, Pastor Rick Warren and thousands of people from his congregation at Saddleback Church started a journey to transform their lives. The result: 15,000 people lost over 260,000 pounds in the first year. But the changes in people's lives went far beyond the pounds they lost.

Feast on Something Bigger Than a Fad *The Daniel Plan: 40 Days to a Healthier Life* by Rick Warren, Dr. Daniel Amen, and Dr. Mark Hyman is far more than a diet plan. It is an appetizing approach to achieving a healthy lifestyle where people are encouraged to get healthier together by optimizing the key five essentials of faith, food, fitness, focus, and friends.

Unlike thousands of other books on the market, this book is not about a new diet fad, guilt-driven gym sessions, or shame-driven fasts. Nor is it a "do it all now" approach. *The Daniel Plan* shows you how focusing on the powerful combination of the key essentials can change your life forever . . . one choice at a time.

The concepts in this book will encourage you to deepen your relationship with God and develop a community of supportive friends who will encourage you to make healthy choices each and every day. The result for you: gradual changes that transform your life inside and out.

Available in stores and online!

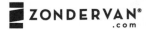

ZONDERVAN®
.com

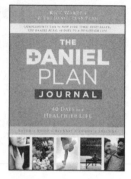
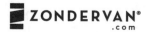

⊞DANIELPLAN

The Daniel Plan Cookbook

Healthy Eating for Life

Rick Warren D. Min., Mark Hyman M.D. and Daniel Amen M.D.

100 DELICIOUS WAYS TO TRANSFORM YOU FROM THE INSIDE OUT

Eating The Daniel Plan way is not only healthy and wholesome; it is the revolutionary program you need to boost your energy and kick start your metabolism. This cookbook is filled with easy-to-prepare recipes based on The Daniel Plan plate, encouraging you to eat life-giving, nutritionally packed whole foods.

Including practical tips, important food facts, and inspiration from The Daniel Plan signature chefs, this book gives you the freedom to choose from a variety of delicious options to create your weekly menu.

Invite your family and friends to join you around the table as you welcome healthy cooking into your kitchen.

Available in stores and online!

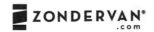

⁑DANIELPLAN

The Daniel Plan Study Guide with DVD

40 Days to a Healthier Life

Rick Warren, Daniel Amen M.D., Mark Hyman M.D.

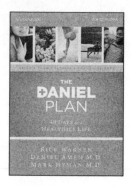

A companion to the *#1 New York Times* bestseller, The Daniel Plan, this six-session video-based, small group study from Rick Warren, Dr. Daniel Amen, and Dr. Mark Hyman is centered on five essentials that will guarantee success in your health journey: faith, food, fitness, focus, and friends.

With assistance from medical and fitness experts, Pastor Rick Warren and thousands of people from his congregation started on a journey to transform their own lives. It's called *The Daniel Plan* and it works for on simple reason: God designed your body to be healthy and vibrant and he provided everything you need to thrive and live an abundant life.

This small group study is a vital component of *The Daniel Plan* because it bakes in the community aspect to its innovative approach to health. As Dr. Mark Hymen says, "community is the medicine" for healthy living.

The Daniel Plan small group study teaches simple ways to incorporate healthy choices into your current lifestyle. This study guide includes Bible study, video discussion questions and notes, practical food and fitness tips to keep you on track each week, and much more.

Session Titles:

- *Faith:* Nurturing Your Soul
- *Food:* Enjoying God's Abundance
- *Fitness:* Strengthening Your Body
- *Focus:* Renewing Your Mind
- *Friends:* Encouraging Each Other
- Living the Lifestyle

Available in stores and online!

◤ ZONDERVAN®
.com